CARING: AN ESSENTIAL HUMAN NEED

Proceedings of Three National Caring Conferences

Madeleine M. Leininger, R.N., Ph.D., LhD., F.A.A.N.
Editor and Author

The World of Caring

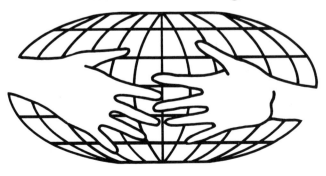

Cover Design by Anthony Frizano

Printed in the United States of America.

ISBN No. 0-913590-83-5

Library of Congress No. 81-51722

Caring is the essence of nursing and the unique and unifying focus of the profession.

—Leininger

Acknowledgments

I wish to gratefully acknowledge all the individuals who have contributed these papers to the Proceedings of the past three National Caring Conferences. These original papers contain some substantive ideas, theories, and research findings to advance the body of knowledge regarding the subject of care and caring. These papers are shared with our interested colleagues to *build upon* this developing baseline of knowledge on caring and to stimulate further theoretical, teaching, and research ideas. Recognition should be made to the source of these ideas from the authors. This rich historical, philosophical, and epistemological content is bound to create a new thrust and excitement about studying caring phenomenon, and especially from cross-cultural viewpoints. For caring remains the essence of nursing and the golden nugget yet to be fully uncovered in professional and academic fields.

I want to acknowledge several nurse leaders who assisted with the planning and implementing of the three National Caring Conferences from 1978 through 1980. These Conferences have been highly successful and have provided a major breakthrough in nursing and the social sciences on caring phenomenon, and I attribute this success to the active support and interest of such nurse leaders as Em Bevis, Joyceen Boyle, Jody Glittenberg, Joyce Murray, Marilyn Ray, Jean Watson, and Darlene Meservy. All were enormously helpful in working with me as Chairwoman to organize and implement each Conference. Darlene Meservy and the secretarial staff of the Division of Continuing Education, College of Nursing of the University of Utah, helped to coordinate activities for the Conferences. Thus, to the nursing leaders, contributors of papers, and coordinators, I am most grateful and appreciative to all. Without such help, cooperation, and stimulation from many colleagues, this successful venture in the discovery of care/caring for research, teaching and practice would not have been possible.

Madeleine Leininger, R.N., Ph.D., Lh.D., F.A.A.N.
Chairwoman, Editor, and Author-Contributor
of the Three National Caring Conferences,
1978, 1979, 1980

Foreword

A series of interesting historical events led to the development of the National Caring Conferences of which this Proceeding contains the first three annual sessions. During the 1976 American Nurses Convention in New Jersey, Dr. Jody Glittenberg and I presented a program on the general subject of caring as the essence of nursing. We found many nurses in attendance were enthusiastic and eager to address the concept of caring as important to nursing. In subsequent communications, these nurses stated: "Isn't it strange that I have attended these ANA conventions for many years, but this is the *first* time I have heard nurses talk directly about caring as the essence of nursing. It seems that we have talked about everything else but caring attitudes and activities." Another recent graduate said, "This is the first time I have ever heard nurses talk about caring or care as related to nursing care. I had nothing like these concepts in my nursing program, and yet they make sense and seem so logical and essential to nursing. In our classes we were taught about curing medical diseases, understanding medical diagnostic techniques, and everything but caring. Thank you for putting caring into nursing care." These and other comments reaffirmed my belief that nurses would focus on caring and its importance in giving nursing care to people if they had some substantive concepts about caring. The nursing students seemed eager to learn about caring if faculty would address the subject.

My early work on cross-cultural caring done in the Eastern Highlands of New Guinea in 1960-62 was the first comparative study focused (in part) on caring phenomenon. This work made me realize the paucity of knowledge about caring and the limited research on the subject. Since then, I have been involved in the study of cultures regarding caring and social structure, and saw the need for the National Caring conferences for nurses and others interested in caring.

Another major factor that led to the National Caring Conferences and the study of the caring phenomenon was the highly positive response of nursing students to special lectures and seminars on caring I had given over the last 16 years while teaching at the Universities of Colorado, Washington, and Utah. These students seemed to come alive whenever caring ideas, theories, or research areas were discussed with them, and especially from a cross-cultural perspective. But with the limited articles and research studies on caring and its relationship to nursing, the students had a difficult time sustaining their interest; and only a few faculty would discuss caring as well, as most of them concentrated on medical diseases and curing. Care was, therefore, the unknown phenomenon that needed to be explicated, analyzed, and used in nursing care as the distinct essence and unifying focus for the nursing profession.

When plans began to take shape for the National Caring Conferences, I was pleased that several nurse leaders such as Em Bevis, Jean Watson, Marilyn Ray, and another colleague, Ann Hyde, were eager for in-depth exchanges on the subject. These colleagues became active supporters for the National Caring Conferences which began in 1978. Thus, several important historical events contributed to my initial work and leadership to make caring a central focus of nursing research and practice, and to establish National Caring Conferences in this country and abroad.

Encouragingly, there are plans to continue with these yearly National Conferences in the future, and to build upon the previous conferences. The plan is to hold the National Conferences in different places in the United States to stimulate national interest in theoretical, clinical, and research studies related to caring and nursing care. The first three conferences were held at the University of Utah in Salt Lake City. They were of high caliber and had participants with multidisciplinary interests, but predominantly nursing and anthropological backgrounds. These colleagues were genuinely interested in advancing ideas on the theory of and in systematically studying caring as well as identifying therapeutic caring practices. Unfortunately, the number of nurses who have conducted studies focused specifically on components or phenomena of caring are few; and so the research and theory will remain a major emphasis for the National Conferences in the future.

Essentially, the National Conferences have been directed toward these major goals:

1) Identification of major philosophical, epistemological, and professional dimensions of caring to advance the body of knowledge that constitutes nursing, and to help other disciplines use caring knowledge in human relationships.
2) Explication of the nature, scope, functions, and structure of care and its relationship to nursing care.
3) Explication of the major components, processes, and patterns of care or caring in relationship to nursing care from a transcultural nursing perspective.
4) Stimulation of nurses and others to systematically investigate care and caring and to share their findings with other interested colleagues.

Unlike many national meetings in nursing, these conferences were in-depth "think-tank" theory and research sharing sessions designed to explore scholarly ideas about caring. The theoretical, research, and clinical aspects of caring have been a central focus of each conference. The participants have met this challenge and remain committed to advance a body of knowledge in nursing about caring. Social scientists and key nurse leaders served as gadflies to sharpen the thinking of the group and to advance ideas beyond local ethnocentric viewpoints. Many nurses who had already participated in the past seven National Transcultural Nursing Conferences were among the most active discussants, and they could use the cross-cultural content for the debates and to explicate caring ideas. This analytical approach to explicate theoretical ideas on caring was crucial to advance ideas about care phenomena. Thus the participants questioned, theorized, and predicted outcomes of caring for nurses, and for use by other disciplines interested in caring. Unfortunately, many of the productive discussions about caring could not be included in this document, but these original papers remain as historical, theoretical, research, and practice documents for future researchers to build upon.

As a consequence of the three National Caring Conferences, there is a growing cadre of nurse scholars and other colleagues who are eager to share, learn, refine, and develop caring content for nursing and for other multidisciplinary uses. The multidisciplinary exchanges were an important outcome of the conferences. For many nurses it was their "scholarship food". Several nurses said to me: "These conferences are unquestionably helping me develop my professional knowledge and interests." Most importantly, the following trends have clearly become evident from the National Conferences:

1) There is definitely more interest and more writings by nurses on the subject of care and caring than in the past, and from all indications, one can predict that more nurses will be writing and doing research on caring in the future.
2) There are several students in master and doctoral programs in nursing eager to study caring behaviors, processes, and outcomes if they can find faculty knowledgeable enough to guide their work on caring. These students seem avid to shift their research from the study of medical diseases, symptoms, and curing to the study of various aspects of caring and its relationship to nursing care.
3) The importance of caring as the heart or central and unifying focus of nursing is *now* being mentioned by nursing leaders at national meetings. Prior to the mid-1970s, there had been virtually no specific focus on caring phenomena and its relationship to nursing care. Instead, topics at most national meetings were about nurse shortages, unions, economic welfare, legislation, and entry into professional practice and related concerns. There was nothing about the sources of caring knowledge and how caring might distinguish nursing from other disciplines.
4) More nursing faculty are now trying to teach ideas about caring phenomena and to encourage research studies on this subject.
5) Other health disciplines, such as physicians, psychologists, and anthropologists, are also becoming interested in caring behaviors and activities.

In general, there is a cultural movement focusing on caring phenomena in nursing which is diffusing within and outside the discipline. This movement reflects a new (or renewed) interest in the unknown dimension of care and its relationship to nursing care. It is making us realize how much there is yet to learn about care and caring. Likewise, business and public establishments are speaking about caring services. But more specific to nursing, there is a critical need to establish caring as our *central and unique focus of the discipline.* Scientific and humanistic caring knowledge with related clinical skills could greatly advance the profession and help the public more fully understand nurses' contributions to society. The original content in this book, plus other writings and research on the subject of caring, should help nurses to value and know the concept of caring. It should stimulate nurses to make caring the central and dominant domain of nursing and to pursue further research on caring. It should help to clarify and reduce current ambiguities about such frequently heard questions from students and professional nurses as, "What is nursing?" "What is nursing about?" "How is nursing different from medicine?" In time, I hope we will be able to establish a scientific and humanistic body of knowledge with practices related to generic caring and nursing care which will be nursing's distinctive contribution to society.

As the initiator and chairwoman of these National Caring Conferences, it has been most encouraging to see the above developments transpire, and especially to see nurses excited to discuss and focus on the concept of caring. Already these Conferences are having an influence upon nursing leaders, students, and other colleagues. Since the National Caring and Transcultural Nursing Conferences have been initiated during the last decade, leadership is now needed to help nurses learn more about caring, and nursing care phenomena. Furthermore, the nursing profession should sponsor and financially support future national and international conferences on caring. Such local, regional, and national conferences are essential to explicate cultural, intellectual, and clinical ideas on caring and nursing care dimensions. The motto of, "Caring is the essence of nursing and the unique and unifying focus of the profession", and the logo should serve as key referent and symbolic guides for the future. The cross-cultural aspects of caring will be a goal for transcultural nurse specialists who are prepared in anthropology and nursing through graduate study.

In summary, I believe an enlightened era in nursing has occurred in which some highly promising and new areas of research, teaching, and practice have been launched related to caring and nursing care. Caring, I believe, is the *sine qua non* of the nursing profession which can make nursing respected, recognized, and a distinct discipline. Understanding scientific and humanistic caring knowledge with clinical skills has the great potential to help individuals know about natural processes and outcomes of human caring, growth, helping processes, and survival. Will the nursing profession take the lead in the pursuit of the study of caring in its fullest dimensions to improve the health and wellbeing of humans? I hope so.

Madeleine Leininger, R.N., Ph.D., Lh.D., F.A.A.N.
Chairwoman, Editor, and Author-Contributor
of the Three National Caring Conferences,
1978, 1979, and 1980.

Author Contributors*

Em Olivia Bevis, R.N., M.A., F.A.A.N.
Professor of Nursing
Head of Savannah Satellite Program
Medical College of Georgia
Savannah, Georgia

Joyceen S. Boyle, R.N., M.P.H.
Predoctoral Nursing Student
College of Nursing
University of Utah
Salt Lake City, Utah

Kathryn G. Gardner, R.N., M.S.
Assistant Nursing Director
Rochester General Hospital
School of Nursing
University of Rochester
Rochester, New York

Delores Ann Gaut, R.N., M.S.N.
Predoctoral Lecturer of Nursing
School of Nursing
University of Washington
Seattle, Washington

Barbara Guthrie, R.N., M.S.N.
Instructor of Nursing
School of Nursing
Duquesne University
Pittsburgh, Pennsylvania

Michael J. Higgins, Ph.D.
Associate Professor of Anthropology
University of Northern Colorado
Greeley, Colorado

Peter Morley, Ph.D.
Associate Professor of Nursing
College of Nursing
University of Utah
Salt Lake City, Utah

Rosemarie Rizzo Parse, R.N., Ph.D.
Professor Nursing
School of Nursing
Duquesne University
Pittsburgh, Pennsylvania

* *Role of Contributors at time papers were presented (1978-1980).*

Marilyn A. Ray, R.N., M.S.N.
Predoctoral Nursing Student
College of Nursing
University of Utah
Salt Lake City, Utah

Joan Uhl, R.N., M.S.
Assistant Professor of Nursing
College of Nursing
University of Utah
Salt Lake City, Utah

Margaret Jean Watson, R.N., M.S.N., Ph.D.
Associate Professor Nursing
School of Nursing
University of Colorado
Denver, Colorado

Erlinda Wheeler, R.N., M.S.
Assistant Professor of Nursing/Clinician,
School of Nursing
University of Rochester
Rochester, New York

Conference Leader and Contributor:

Madeleine M. Leininger, R.N., Lh.D., Ph.D., F.A.A.N.
Dean and Professor of Nursing
Adjunct Professor of Anthropology
College of Nursing
University of Utah
Salt Lake City, Utah.

Conference Coordinator:

Darlene Meservy, R.N., M.P.H.
Assistant Professor of Nursing
College of Nursing
University of Utah
Salt Lake City, Utah

These Conferences were supported, in part, by the Division of Continuing Education, University of Utah, Salt Lake City, Utah.

Table of Contents
of the
THREE NATIONAL CARING CONFERENCES

FIRST NATIONAL CONFERENCE

"THE PHENOMENA AND NATURE OF CARING"
(April 27, 28, 29, 1978, Salt Lake City, Utah)

SECOND NATIONAL CONFERENCE

"ANALYSIS OF CARING BEHAVIORS AND PROCESSES"
(March 22, 23, 1979, Salt Lake City, Utah)

THIRD NATIONAL CONFERENCE

"CHARACTERISTICS AND CLASSIFICATION OF CARING PHENOMENA"

(March 18, 19, 1980, Salt Lake City, Utah)

Part I — 1978

The Phenomena and Nature of Caring
First National Caring
Conference

April 27, 28, 29, 1978
University of Utah
Salt Lake City, Utah

The Phenomenon of Caring: Importance, Research Questions and Theoretical Considerations

1

Madeleine Leininger, R.N., Ph.D., Lh.D., F.A.A.N.

In recent years, a few nurse researchers have directed their work towards theories, models, and research methods to explicate the body of knowledge relevant to the discipline of nursing. Such intellectual activities have been essential and encouraging in order to identify the nature, essence, and domains of inquiry that will help to advance nursing and distinguish the field from other academic and professional disciplines. Much more rigorous work is needed by nurse scholars to achieve this important goal in nursing.

In the identification of domains of inquiry in nursing, it is an interesting and curious fact that there has been very limited systematic and rigorous study regarding the nature and phenomenon of caring by nurse researchers. Although nurses have linguistically said that they *give care* and they talk about nursing care activities, still there has been virtually no systematic investigation of the epistemological, philosophical, linguistic, social, and cultural aspects of caring, and the relationship of care to professional nursing care theory and practice. Furthermore, care *per se* is seldom defined in nursing, and yet it is used regularly as the suffix to nursing.

The purpose of this paper, as introduction to the first National Caring Conference, is to explore some general philosophical, linquistic, cultural, and professional viewpoints, assumptions, questions, and theoretical considerations about caring as the central and unifying domain of inquiry for nursing as a discipline and for professional practices. Studying caring as an area for humanistic and scientific nursing care will also be discussed.

Potential of Caring as a Central and Unifying Domain for Nursing

It has long been the author's position that ***caring*** *is the central and unifying domain for the body of knowledge and practices in nursing,* and a systematic investigation of caring could advance the discipline of nursing and ultimately provide better nursing care to people.[1] I hold that an in-depth knowledge of caring from diverse perspectives and from a historical, philosophical, and epistemological study will enable nurses and other caregivers to know the full nature of care or caring behaviors, patterns, and processes. Most importantly, as nursing moves toward full disciplinary status, it will be essential for nurses to know the nature, scope, and distinguishing features that characterize nursing from other health disciplines. I hold that caring behavior and practices *uniquely* distinguish nursing from the contributions of other disciplines. Thus the critical and essential challenge is for nurses to systematically and rigorously explicate and analyze caring phenomena in depth and breadth, and from a cross-cultural viewpoint.

The importance of caring to the nursing profession and to humanity appears evident, but there are many questions yet to be answered:

1) What is the essential nature of care/caring?
2) How is caring expressed among different cultures in the world?
3) What are the philosophical and epistemological arguments for caring and nursing in human cultures?
4) What is the cultural history of caring in nursing from an anthropological viewpoint?
5) What are the essential generic elements of caring?
6) What is the difference between professional and non-professional caring attributes, processes, and patterns?
7) What characterizes caring patterns and processes in nursing from other disciplines?
8) What are the cross-cultural differences in human caring and professional caring?
9) What does caring for strangers mean?
10) What is the relationship of care to nursing care?
11) What are the categories of care and nursing care?
12) What theories about care or caring offer promise to know caring phenomena and its fullest dimensions? and
13) Why has nursing failed to study the epistemological, philosophical, and cultural aspects of caring as generic to nursing?

When answers to these and other questions become known, a *body of caring science* will evolve to advance nursing knowledge and other professional aspects about care behaviors and processes in nursing.

Undoubtedly, caring has long been expressed by human cultures throughout the history of humankind. Care, I believe, was *essential* for human growth, development, and survival. This anthropological and nursing position makes one pause to consider the importance and significance of caring for the human race and for the lifeways of *homo sapiens* as a species. If this major assumption can be investigated, then nurses and others should give more attention to this phenomena. Such research would be especially pertinent to nursing as a profession since they have laid claim to nursing care for many decades. Caring appears to be an extremely important and generic construct in human services. It appears to be at the heart of all health care services. It is the largely unknown ingredient for helping humankind in wellness, illness, and stressful situations. Why then, has so little attention been given to caring by humanistically-oriented scientists and caregivers? This question is an intriguing one that has yet to be answered, and one which deserves more thought than it has received in the past. It is a question that could lead to many fascinating research lines of inquiry about human behavior in health and illness states.

World View: An Anthropological Approach to Study Care and Caring

During the past decade, I have been active in designing and conceptualizing ways to study caring phenomenon from both nursing and anthropological perspectives.[1,2] The need exists for a broad framework for cross-cultural differences and similarities about patterns, processes, and behaviors related to care and caring. At the same time, a need exists to explore in-depth, the multiple aspects of caring from an anthropological viewpoint, including the cultural, linguistic, and professional practices of nursing as a caring profession. To meet these expectations, I have used an ethnoscientific approach to study the perceptions, cognitions, and actions of a designated group of nurses and clients in different cultures. (Leininger M: unpublished research, 1964-1981.) The ethnonursing context and practices of caring were also studied. It was the world view of the informants that has been extremely helpful to my investigation of caring phenomenon, for this view supports and is closely related to ethnocaring and ethnonursing.

It was Redfield who introduced the term, "world view" to social science many years ago. World view refers to the way individuals or cultures grow, perceive, and know their world about them.[3] This concept should be an integral part of *all* nursing practices, teaching, and research work. The world view approach expects that the nurse would understand the world of the client, and to feel, know, and experience his/her world. The world view means that one tries to get a broad gestalt of another person's lifeways, or a cultural perspective of living. Using this approach, one constantly seeks for insight about many diverse aspects of human living, and yet looks at the unifying values and lifeways of an individual. Sensitivity and attention to the aspects of values and beliefs are important in seeing the world view of another human being, as well as the context in which that individual lives.

In the use of the world view and the ethnoscientific approach to caring, one focuses upon linguistic and daily features of caring from the individual's viewpoint as well as group cultural views about caring. Both the *similarities* and *differences* among individuals as they know, perceive, and experience caring is important. The humanistic and scientific aspects of caring are also identified when a world view approach is used to study caring.

A world view approach is essential to conceptualize paradigms, theories, and models related to holistic caring. Kuhn has discussed the role and importance of paradigms in the evolution of the body of knowledge of a discipline, and he challenges the belief that knowledge and scientific fields have developed through steady and slow increments of knowledge. He believes that science advances through a revolution in which concepts, theories, and research methods are overthrown by new paradigms which are accepted by the majority of scientists in that discipline.[4] It is my position that advances in knowledge occur both by *revolution* and *evolution*. Nurses must be aware of both processes to develop a body of knowledge about caring and nursing care phenomena. Diverse paradigms about caring are therefore important to revolutionize and to help evolve nursing—especially its distinctive features. Paradigms which move beyond local world views to cross-cultural paradigms of caring are essential in order to help nurses discover the universal and specific aspects of caring. Most importantly, world view paradigms are needed to study the humanistic and scientific aspects of caring in broad dimensions.

Ambiguities About Caring

Vagueness and ambiguities about caring by nurses have been evident for many years. Nurses and other health professionals use the terms *care, caring, health care* and *nursing care,* but there is virtually no scientific or humanistic knowledge base for these terms. Moreover, there is divergent professional and social usage about care. The effects or consequences of caring behaviors upon individuals, families, and communities by professional caregivers remains limitedly validated or understood to date. The terms *care, caring* and *nursing care* are often used interchangeably among nurses, and frequently in a loose and non-discriminatory manner in written and verbal discussion. Many divergent ideas are used by nurses when they talk about care in different settings and with different preparation. So when nursing care is used by nurses, ambiguities exist regarding the meaning, function, and therapeutic usage of nursing care.

Further consideration of the linguistic and functional usages of care reveals that *care* and *nursing care* are something which all nurses are expected to know about and to use in practice. The generic use of care and its relationship to nursing care is also unclear in teaching and research. Concepts about caregivers and care recipients remain an area of inquiry, as well as care activities, patterns, and behaviors. Presently, in many schools of nursing, in-depth presentations on the nature of caring behaviors, processes, and patterns remain unexplored. Nursing faculty will speak of *nursing care,* and different ideas about medical care are often discussed. Furthermore, nursing curricula still contain far more content on medical diseases, conditions, and curative treatment regimes than nursing care or caring behaviors.[5] Searching for the essence, nature, expression, and function of caring and its relationship to nursing care remains a major area of investigation. Linguistic, philosophical, and professional usages of care or caring are open areas for teaching and research in nursing. I believe we should not continue to make linguistic usage and professional claims to care and nursing care with so little knowledge about the essential and generic nature of care. Diverse theories and conceptual frameworks (or paradigms) about care/caring would help to explicate caring and care. Again, why such limited attention to caring, when it is claimed by nursing and is of much interest to nurses? It is unfortunate that caring has not been a central theoretical and research area in nursing until very recently. Instead, there are research studies on topics such as time, motion, energy, adaptation, and other concepts. Concepts and theories related to caring appear essential to know and to link with ideas related to nursing care. Thus, it is time to focus on caring in research, teaching, and practice in order to bring credence and legitimacy to a major implied and claimed concept that has been used in nursing for more than 100 years.

Rationale for Studying Caring

To encourage nurse researchers and others to pursue caring research, several major reasons can be offered why this construct appears important to investigate.

First, the construct of ***care** appears critical to human growth, development, and survival for human beings for millions of years.* Caring appears to be the largely unknown ingredient for helping others under the threat of illness in a humanistic and scientific manner. From an anthropological viewpoint, I hold that caring must have been a mode of human action and relatedness from the beginning of humankind. Caring appears to be one of the most human acts and a quality for being human rather than animal-like in behavior. Unfortunately, anthropologists have not explicated caring as essential to human existence; and yet the need seems logical for human survival through the millennia.

One can assume that cultures depended upon care and caring through millions of years for human survival; however, the prehistory and historical aspects of caring have not been identified. How was caring expressed by cultural groups and among individuals? How was caring manifested in the prehistoric days when people lived in changing and precarious environments? What would constitute primitive caring and how would it differ from professional caring today?

I believe that caring was the *critical* and *important factor* that assisted *homo sapiens* through cultural evolution. I believe caring was essential to growth and survival of the race amid a variety of stressful environmental changes. I believe that humanistic caring helped people to live and survive under most adverse and changing environments and in relation to changing economic, political, cultural, and social factors.

A second reason to study care is to explicate caregiver and care recipient roles in various living and survival contexts. Presently, we know little about caregiver and care recipient behaviors as well as the ways care is provided by different nurses and non-nurses in diverse cultures. Caregiving behaviors associated with health and illness must have been important in the prehistoric days as well as today to help people overcome trauma and illness states. Who were the early caregivers and how was care given? Have women always been the principal caregivers? How was care given when environmental catastrophies occurred, such as floods, fires, and hurricanes? In diverse societies, human caring modes must have been as significant in the past as they are today. Caring must also have linked people together in patterns of interdependency. One also wonders if caregivers had status in the past, and if not, why? What status or recognition is given to caregivers today? What historical means do we have to study caregiver and care recipient roles? How did caregiver behavior become culturally constituted with explicit socialization processes in the distant past? These additional questions address important historical and epistemological aspects of care behavior, and cultural patterns, and offer ideas for future research studies.

A third reason for studying caring is to *preserve* and *maintain* this human attribute for current and future human cultures. Today there are multiple forces that appear to be devaluing and demeaning human life such as the lack of respect for human lives through homocides and suicides. There is the depersonalization of humans with technological equipment. And there are multiple economic, political, and legal constraints that daily threaten humans, and reflect a lack of human caring or concern for others. Evidence of war, feuds, violence, and legal threats are other signs of the less caring society in which we live. We need to buttress a caring lifeway to ourselves and others to preserve and maintain human societies. Caring processes, patterns, and expressions might well become extinct if we do not recognize caring and value it in our lives. Without caring, one could speculate that the human race could destroy itself. I believe caring helps to bridge human relatedness, concern, and compassionate help to others. Human care appears to have existed through time and is universal to human existence and helping processes, and therefore, it must be preserved. With the increased use of technology, human caring appears less evident in health and human services, and health professionals such as those in the nursing profession could provide a renewed emphasis on human caring and make known caring attibutes.

A fourth reason for studying caring is that since the beginning of modern professional nursing, the nursing profession has not systematically studied caring in relation to nursing care. Although Florence Nightingale used the term *care,* she never explicated, defined, or discussed its function. Her use of care was often noted in relation to helping people live or survive in their physical or natural environment. To Nightingale, care was related to cleanliness, fresh air, good food, rest, sleep, and exercise.[6] Good health care seemed synonomous with good health habits and a healthy environment. According to Nightingale, the goal or task of nursing is "to put the patient in the best condition for nature to act upon him."[7] Her ideas were primarily on environmental and physical care, especially when sick. These ideas were important for nursing and its evolution as a profession, but care *per se* was not defined.

Definition of Care/Caring

Since the days of Florence Nightingale, the word *care* has been used in nursing as a verb, as in *to be cared for, caring for others,* or *to manifest care* with concern, compassion and interested in another human being. Care and caring appear to have multiple conceptualizations and characterizations. Although care has a common and recurrent usage by nurses, definitions of care are needed to include strangers who give care by comfort, alleviation of distress, and other human ways. While definitions of *nursing care* can be found in the literature, there are few that define the *generic concept of care.* For example, in Henderson's work (frequently used by nurses), she speaks of nursing and implies care activities:[8]

> ...Nursing is primarily helping people (sick or well) in the performance of those activities contributing to health, or its recovery (or to a peaceful death) that they would perform unaided if they had the necessary strength, will, or knowledge.

For heuristic purposes, I define ***care/caring*** *in a generic sense as those assistive, supportive, or facilitative acts toward or for another individual or group* with evident or anticipated needs to ameliorate or improve a human condition or lifeway. I define ***professional caring*** as those cognitive and culturally learned action behaviors, techniques, processes, or patterns that enable (or help) an individual, family, or community to improve or maintain a favorably healthy condition or lifeway. And finally, I define ***professional nursing care*** *as those cognitively learned humanistic and scientific modes of helping or enabling an individual, family, or community to receive personalized services* through specific culturally defined or ascribed modes of caring processes, techniques, and patterns to improve or maintain a favorably healthy condition for life or death.[9]

In the above definitions, one will note the emphasis is on *helpful* and *enabling* activities of individuals, social, and community groups based upon culturally defined, ascribed, or sanctioned modes of helping people. I believe that caring acts can be culturally identified through the beliefs, values, and practices of cultural groups. From a cross-cultural study of caring behaviors, one can then identify what caring acts, processes, and techniques are culturally specific, and those that are universal. Other theoretical and philosophical positions will be discussed later with the focus on discovering transcultural nursing care phenomenon.

In Mayeroff's work, he speaks about caring with some general attributes:[10]

> ...Caring is the antithesis of simply using the other person to satisfy one's needs. The meaning of caring I want to suggest is not to be confused with such meanings as wishing well, liking, comforting and maintaining, or simply having an interest in what happens to another. Also, it is not an isolated feeling or a momentary relationship, nor is it simply a matter of wanting to care for some person. Caring, as helping another grow and actualize himself, is a process, a way of relating to someone that involves *development,* in the same way that friendship can only emerge through mutual trust and a deepening and qualitative transformation of the relationship.

Rollo May also offered some ideas about care in his discussion about man living and relating to the world in which he lives:[11]

> ...Care is the necessary source of eros, the source of human tenderness...Care is given power by nature's sense of pain; if we do not care for ourselves we are hurt...
>
> ...In care one must by involvement with the objective fact, do something about the situation; one must make some decisions. This is where care brings love and will together...

From cursory review of the philosophy and the social, biological, and health science literature, the terms *care* and *caring for others* are frequently used. Many diverse ideas are associated with care, such as being used analogously with love, tenderness, compassion, and empathy. Accordingly, in the dictionary the verbs *care, caring,* and *cared* mean: to have an interest in, to be concerned for, to provide or look after, and to be disposed to help others.[12] One could then infer that *to not care* for someone would reflect indifference, antipathy, disregard for another, lack of attention, or no interest in helping another human being. Noncaring behaviors are of equal interest to study.

During the past decade I have found in studying nearly 30 world cultures through interviews, structured questionnaire guides, literature sources, and direct observations, that there are many concepts associated with care or caring. Intercultural variations clearly exist with no universal ethnoscience definition or social usage of care by cultural representatives. While the data are still under analysis and being checked for validation of what informants *said* with the *actual* cultural practices, the following constructs are associated closely with care/caring (varying in cultural usage with respect to which terms are used in different cultures): support, tenderness, touch, compassion, empathy, stress alleviation, presence, loving acts, comfort, direct and indirect helping behaviors, enabling, facilitating, nurturance, succorance, surveillance, protection, restoration, instructive acts, coping, concern, interest in, trusting, and need fulfillment.[9] With each of these constructs, there are many embedded ideas associated with the concepts of care or caring. And there are some constructs that may not be found in designated cultures. For example, the nurse as a caregiver is not permitted by cultural rules to touch a patient in the Yap culture. How would an Anglo-American nurse provide care to the Yap people in the Micronesian cultural area? Many extremely fascinating data are coming from my investigation, which should throw new light on old conceptualizations of nursing care and the need to use transcultural caring knowledge in culturally specific ways.

Some Assumptions and Beliefs About Human Caring

In pursuit of knowing the nature of humanistic and scientific caring, and based upon my preliminary research findings, I have identified several assumptions to guide nurses' deliberations about caring. The following assumptions may challenge nurses to discover in depth the phenomenon of caring:

1) Human caring is a universal phenomenon, but the expressions, processes, and patterns vary among cultures.
2) Every nursing care situation has transcultural caring behaviors, needs, and implications.
3) Caring acts and processes are essential for human development, growth, and survival.
4) Caring should be considered the essence and unifying intellectual and practice dimension of professional nursing.
5) Caring has biophysical, psychological, cultural, social, and environmental dimensions which can be studied, and practices to provide holistic care to people.
6) Transcultural caring behaviors, forms, and processes have yet to be verified from diverse cultures; when this body of knowledge is procurred, it has the potential to revolutionize present-day nursing practices.
7) To provide therapeutic nursing care, the nurse should have knowledge of caring values, beliefs, and practices of the client(s).
8) Caring behaviors and functions vary with social structure features of any designed culture.
9) The identification of universal and non-universal folk and professional caring behaviors, beliefs, and practices will be important to advance the body of nursing knowledge.
10) Differences exist between the essence and essential features of caring and curing behaviors and processes.
11) There can be no curing without caring, but there may be caring without curing.

Some Theoretical Statements and Hypotheses About Caring

The following theoretical statements or hypotheses are offered to stimulate research studies on caring behaviors, processes, and patterns. A few nurses are already investigating aspects of these hypotheses.[9]

1) Intercultural differences in beliefs, values, and practices of caring would reflect differences in nursing care practices.
2) Self-care practices will be valued and practiced in cultures that value individualism and independence in social structure features, whereas group care practice will be valued and practiced in cultures where interdependency and high individualism *is not* espoused.
3) Congruence between caregiver and care recipient's behaviors and goals is important for therapeutic practices to occur.
4) The greater the differences between folk caring values and professional caring values, the greater the signs of cultural conflict and stresses between professional caregivers and non-professional care receivers.
5) Technological caring acts, techniques, and practices differ in cultures and have different outcomes for health and nursing care practices.

6) The greater the efforts of professional nurses to blend the folk caring practices with professional care practices, the greater the signs of clients' satisfactions.
7) The nurse as a professional caregiver may produce unfavorable stresses and conflicts with the client due to lack of knowledge about cultural beliefs, values, and practices of caring.
8) Symbolic forms of nursing care behaviors have referent meanings in different cultural groups and necessitate that nurses study the meaning and functions of symbols in cultures to give efficacious nursing care.
9) The greater the signs of technological caregiving, the less signs of interpersonal care manifestations.
10) Caring behaviors and patterns are closely linked to social structure features.

A Conceptual Model for Studying Transcultural Nursing Care Theories and Practices

During this time I have been investigating the definitions, nature, and scope of the care and caring, using an ethnoscientific approach. (Leininger M: unpublished data, 1964-1981.) The study of the cultural usages, meanings, and functions of caring in different cultures appears closely related to the social structure and cultural beliefs of people. Essentially, my research is focused on explicating and studying caring phenomenon from different cultural viewpoints. A body of ethnocaring knowledge is being sought. I am interested in how people perceive, know, and experience caring behaviors in different cultures so that nurses can use this knowledge in providing both cultural-specific or cultural-universal nursing care practices. *The ultimate goal is to improve health care to people.* Transcultural health care should become more manifest, along with the new generation of nursing care theories and practices.

To date, approximately 30 cultures have been studied by direct interviews, structured questionnaires, library data, and direct observations focused upon beliefs and practices related to caring. From these data, a taxonomy of caring constructs, theories, and hypotheses are being developed. The conceptual framework is offered in Figure 1.1.[9] In the model one can identify a dynamic process to cross-cultural caring phenomenon. It is a process model to show how the knowledge on caring is obtained and validated. On the left side of the model, Phase I, are the major sources from which I derived ethnocaring data that have been identified, namely, by doing an ethnography (or lifeways of the societies), studying the social structure features, cultural values, and in identifying the health-illness caring behaviors and practices in a designated culture. Phase I is followed by Phase II, which focuses upon the identification of the major enthnocaring constructs from data obtained from Phase I domains, and examples of these constructs are offered. Several subsets of ideas are found within each construct. These constructs have been prioritized and defined by the people. Phase III reflects the next step in ethnocare study by analyzing the data and developing theories that will be tested in

FIGURE 1.1

LEININGER'S CONCEPTUAL AND THEORY-GENERATING MODEL TO STUDY TRANSCULTURAL AND ETHNOCARING CONSTRUCTS*

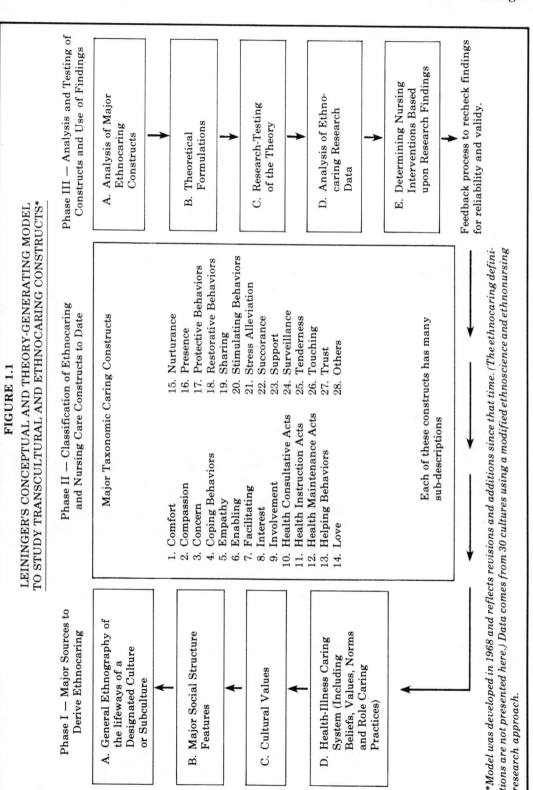

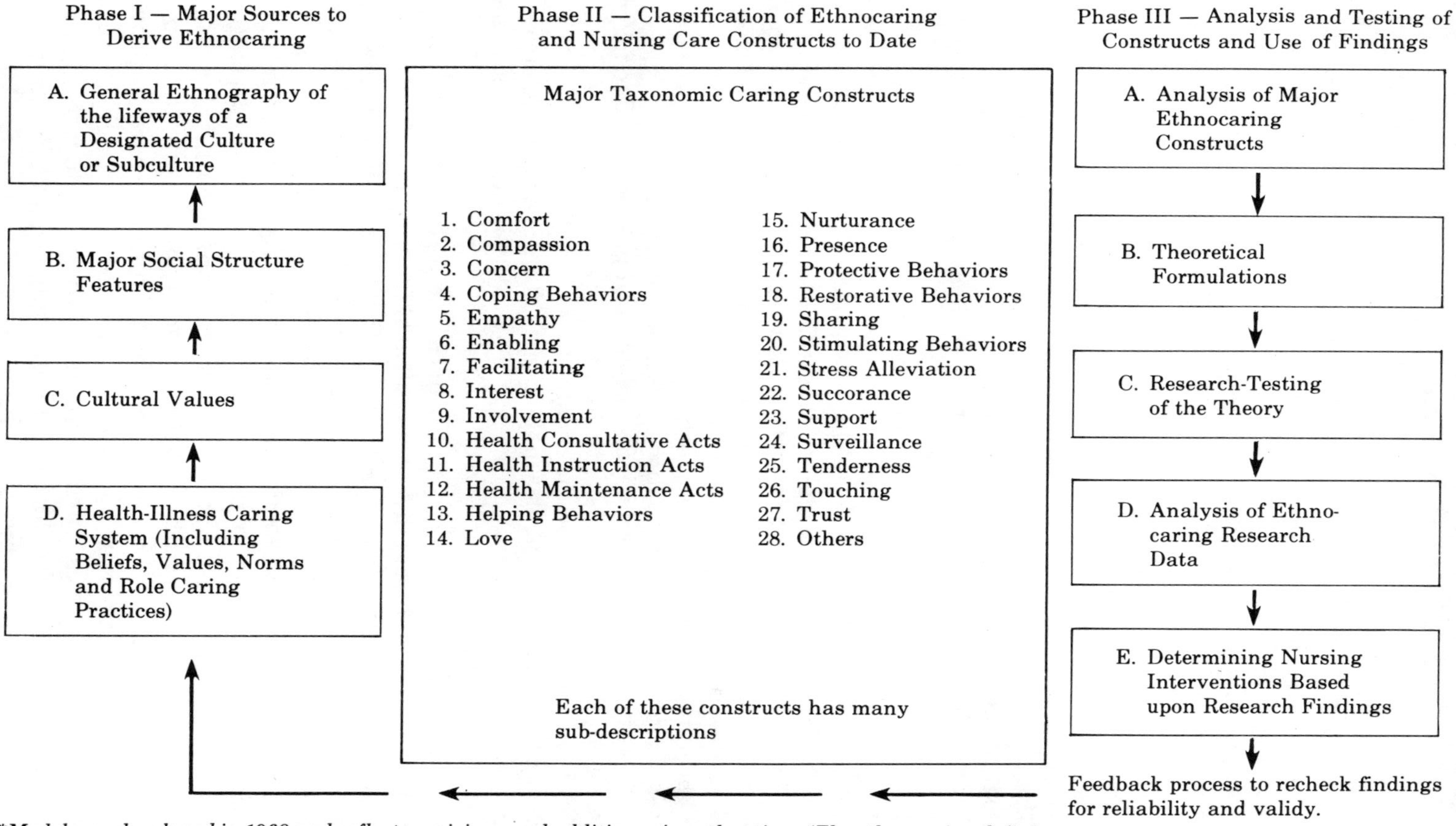

**Model was developed in 1968 and reflects revisions and additions since that time. (The ethnocaring definitions are not presented here.) Data comes from 30 cultures using a modified ethnoscience and ethnonursing research approach.*

subsequent research. The model also shows ways to recycle findings to check for reliability and validity of the data.

From the research work to date, there are several common principles or guidelines which have become evident and could be used to help nurses focus on and further refine caring behaviors and processes. They are as follows:

1) Caring behaviors and processes can be identified in cultures to help guide nursing care decisions and actions.
2) Caring behaviors appear closely related to the social structure features of designated cultures and can help to predict nursing care behaviors of the cultural groups.
3) Caring rituals may be therapeutic and non-therapeutic depending upon how closely the caregiver links activities with cultural values and beliefs.
4) Caring behaviors vary transculturally in priorities, expressions, and need satisfactions.
5) Westernized nurses tend to rely heavily on technological and psychophysiological stress alleviation activities to help clients; whereas nurses in non-Westernized cultures tend to rely more frequently on non-technological and more sociocultural expressions of behaviors.
6) Caring behaviors appear more important than curing in recovery of clients, but receive less economic and social reward than curing by physicians.
7) Efficacious caring tends to be humanistically oriented and reflects professional care concepts of concern, compassion, stress alleviation, nurturance, comfort, and protection, and especially by female caregivers.
8) Caring behaviors have important symbolic referents which need to be identified and used in therapeutic care practices.
9) Caregiving and care receiving behaviors require signs of reciprocal behavior satisfactions for such activities to continue over time.
10) Professional nursing care values, beliefs, and practices tend to follow more medical and curing model attributes in the United States than caring attributes as perceived by the clients.
11) Self-care is gaining emphasis in the United States, but has less credence and relevance in other parts of the world—especially non-Western cultures—where other care is emphasized.

Such preliminary findings (and others yet to be identified) indicate the enormously rich data found in a cross-cultural focus on caring. From such data come guides to help nurses and others give therapeutic care. Knowledge of the values, beliefs, and practices of a culture regarding caring opens the door to culture-specific care and universal caring practices. The close interrelationships of care, culture, and social structure is clearly apparent from my cross-cultural work on caring behaviors, patterns, and processes. It appears essential that professional nurses know variations in cultural caring, and the ways caring is linked with specific value systems. Future and ongoing research on caring and its relationship to nursing care appears highly promising and encouraging. I believe a new breakthrough in nursing has occurred with the focus on caring and its relationship to nursing and health care practices. Nurses should build upon such research findings, and other theories and research studies of caring.

In summary, caring should be the central, critical, and unifying domain and focus for nursing care knowledge. The generic construct of caring is essential to explicate nursing. The possibilities for developing a scientific and humanistic body of nursing knowledge related to caring appears favorable. However, too many nurses are still following medicine and focusing on their medical model of diagnosing and curing largely physical illnesses, rather than on the caring phenomenon. The transcultural nursing approach provides a highly promising mode for studying universal and non-universal aspects of caring in all areas of nursing for all cultures. This knowledge can then be linked to nursing care practices and to make essential changes for a humanistic and scientific body of caring knowledge. This contribution will not only serve nursing, but other disciplines and human groups. I believe we are on the threshold of some new discoveries in nursing that will make nursing's contribution visible, substantive, and distinctive in the near future.

References

1. Leininger M: Caring: The Essence and Central Focus of Nursing. American Nurses' Foundation (Nursing Research Report), Vol 12, No 1, February 1977, p 2.
2. Leininger M: Towards Conceptualization of Transcultural Health Care Systems: Concepts and a Model. In Health Care Dimensions, Philadelphia, FA Davis Co., 1976.
3. Redfield R: The Little Community. Chicago, University of Chicago Press, 1957.
4. Kuhn TS: The Structure of Scientific Revolutions. Chicago, University of Chicago Press, 1970.
5. Leininger M: Review of Large Sample of Baccalaureate and Master Degree Programs for NLN Board of Review from 1976-79.
6. Nightingale F: Notes on Nursing. New York, Dover Publications, 1969.
7. Nightingale F: Notes on Nursing: What It Is and What It Is Not. Philadelphia, B Lippincott, 1964, p 3.
8. Henderson V, Nite G: Principles and Practice of Nursing. New York, Macmillan Publishing Co, Inc, 6th ed, 1978.
9. Leininger M: Transcultural Nursing Concepts, Theories, and Practices. New York, John Wiley and Sons, 1978, p 35-38, 39.
10. Mayeroff M: On Caring. New York, Harper & Row Publishers, 1971, p 1.
11. May R: Love and well. New York, Norton, 1969, pp 286-8.
12. Oxford English Dictionary, p 339.

Conceptual Analysis of *Caring*: Research Method

2

Delores Ann Gaut, R.N., M.S.N.

Introduction: Status and Problem

Examination of the periods of growth in the history of nursing education permits one to identify the expressions, slogans, and concepts that have helped to shape educational policies in nursing. One such term or concept gaining in popularity among nurses is that of *caring*. Certainly the term is not new to nurses. From the writings of Florence Nightingale to present-day authors, caring has held a position of unwavering importance, even though the meanings inherent in the term have at best only been alluded to.

Early writers had a vision of nursing and nurse education that embraced a number of enduring beliefs—among them the belief that although nursing was indeed an art and a science, the real depth of nursing could only be known through the ideals of love, sympathy, knowledge, and culture.[1] Today, definitions of nursing might still include the notion of nursing as an art and a science, but they will also undoubtedly include some reference to caring as an essential component of the process of nursing.

Because nurses and nurse educators have been dependent upon the social sciences for much of their knowledge about human behavior, discourses about caring stem in large part from the writings of philosophers and social scientists such as Buber,[2] Erikson,[3] Jourard,[4] Rogers,[5] and Mayeroff.[6] Following the lead of theorists, nurse educators called for a change in nursing school curriculum that would emphasize the importance of human relationships in nursing. For writers like Orlando,[7] Peplau[8] and Travelbee,[9] the helping relationship between the nurse and the patient was not only an adjunct to medical treatment, but was to be considered a direct therapeutic tool to bring about healing. Henderson, writing in the 1960s, departed from the widely accepted objective stance of nurse to patient and asked the nurse to understand and care for the patient in a new way—as she put it, "to get inside his skin...to give of self."[10]

Emphasis on the relationship between nurse and patient threw new light on the enlarging role of the nurse, and caring took on even greater importance. The nursing profession took positive steps toward defining the role of the nurse in 1965, when the American Nurses' Association identified the essential components of nursing as, "care, cure, and coordination."[11] The components of cure and coordination were discussed in detail. The caring aspect was limited to identifying that somehow caring was to be more than the concept of "to take care of", as in traditional physical care; it was also to include "to care for and care about."[11] Somewhere between *to take care of* and *to care about* there was a qualitative difference that once achieved would enhance both the *caring of* and *caring for.*

The distinction between the two senses of caring is not readily obvious, nor does *taking care of* necessarily imply *caring for.* In analyzing such a statement, one might become convinced that there was a reliance on jargon just to make a point. In other words, the use of phrases such as *to take care of* and *to care for* have a familiar and even authoritative ring to them, but without further clarification both statements remain vague. Could it be possible that *caring* is really nothing more than a slogan to provide a rallying point for nurses involved in a movement toward professionalism and role identification? It is possible that caring is a key idea in many nursing slogans, but at the same time, it seems to be found more and more in nursing literature as a principle for action, a case in point for arguments, and in certain instances a doctrine for belief.

My review of the recent nursing literature indicated that the use of the concept of caring has grown rapidly since the 1960s. Nursing textbooks, nursing journals, statements of philosophy in schools of nursing, and even behavioral student objectives in some way referred to caring. A few examples might illustrate my point. In one textbook nursing is defined as a caring process in which one shows "compassionate concern for the individual."[12] A statement of belief from the philosophy of a school of nursing defines caring as "the acceptance of responsibility for another person when assistance is needed."[13] In describing the components of nursing, an educator included nurturance, defined as "a caring relationship which fosters reciprocal giving and receiving among those involved in the relationship."[14]

These examples are just a few instances of the extent to which caring has permeated the discourse on nursing. But what is it about *caring* that makes it so usable? Is it a concept through which practices and policies can be justified, or is it a vague and ambiguous term referring to a quality that cannot be measured because it has too many meanings to have any one meaning? To begin, let me distinguish between slogans and justification, and then discuss the analysis of a concept.

Slogans, according to Scheffler, are unsystematic, popular sayings that are to be repeated reassuringly, with little thought.[15] Slogans have no standard form and make no claim to facilitate discourses or to explain the meanings of terms. Slogans provide rallying points for key ideas and attitudes of movements and with the passage of time tend to assume the tone of doctrine and be used in argument.[15] So it might be with *caring.* The term can now be found used indiscriminately and without definition in numerous statements about nursing and nurse education. To seek out possible definitions of caring, it would be important to evaluate the caring slogans both as straightforward assertions and as symbols of a social movement in nursing.

Justification, however, is quite different from the use of slogans. Questions of justification are questions about the acceptability of statements made. To justify a statement or policy one asks, "What reasons do we have for accepting this as true?" The justification relies on a certain principle or set of principles which do the justifying.[16] For example, we justify claims of factual knowledge by means of empirical proof; we cite evidence. We justify claims of mathematical truth by proof dependent on conformity to principles. And we justify moral approval or disapproval by reference to ethical principles.[17] Justification involves at least an implicit reference to some standards or norms which serve as principles. At this point the question might be asked, "Is caring in fact such a principle or norm by which decisions, policies, and practices in nursing are justified?" Assuming a positive reply, then one necessarily looks for definitions of caring that would adequately explicate what is intended by the term in the language of common sense and of science. Reviews of the philosophical literature have not revealed such definitions. The problem then seems to be that the concept of caring, initially used in nursing as a slogan, has through time and increased use been given the role of a justifying principle or norm for various statements and policies about nursing and nurse education, with little explication of the meaning or meanings of the concept.

In speaking of the definition of a term I do not mean to imply that there will be a single clear and precise meaning, but rather that the term being defined has a family of meanings, related and broad in scope. The central notion of *definition,* then, is setting forth the meanings of a word. At this point analytic philosophy becomes valuable, for a major technique of analysis is to try to formulate precisely the meanings of terms that are of special interest.[17]

Though no one simple description of philosophical analysis prevails today, the philosophers adopting the theory and methods of Wittgenstein seem especially interested in addressing the question of justification. In search of the "principle of verifiability," the analyst transforms the traditional question "What does X mean?" into "What would you do to recognize an instance of X?"[18] For my purposes, the question would be "What must be true to say that X is caring for S?" To begin to answer, I will attempt to analyze the concept of caring.

Analysis of a concept is the description of its use. Insofar as philosophy is analytic, it is primarily concerned with clarification of concepts and their relations. Although conceptual analysis often appears to be discourse about discourse, the questions are asked in terms of concepts to be analyzed and patterns of thinking to be clarified. When someone learns a concept, he learns a rule of behavior in the use of language. Such rules are open, allow for flexibility, and often require clarification. The purpose of studying a concept, then, is to refine a concept already understood in order to arrive at an extended definition.[19] In philosophy, the technique of explication has been developed as an alternative to definition. In seeking to explicate a term, philosophers try to capture as much of the meaning as they can precisely characterize.[20]

Like a definition, an analysis is always a formulation of meaning, but it is also more than that. Analysis of a concept attempts to describe when the concept applies and when it does not, how its nuances include one to think one way or another when using it, and the differences of meaning it receives in different contexts.[19] Approaching the analysis of *caring,* I ask, "How does the idea of caring function in thought? How does it give structure to thinking and acting? What are caring activities, what are not, and why?" Answering those kinds of questions might begin to reveal what role the concept actually plays in thinking as well as in discourse.

Because the philosophical method deals with problems concerned with formulating, analyzing, and to some extent justifying educational statements and policies, I intend to use in this study, philosophical analysis as a mode of inquiry. The purpose of such study will be to search for a strong definition or explication of caring. The definition will include not only what would count as caring, but also noncaring. I am aware that the application of philosophical methods to education or nurse education is not to hold forth an answer for the practical difficulties encountered in the discipline. But I do believe that it is essential for nursing and nurse educators to understand the ways in which nurses formulate beliefs, arguments, assumptions, and to make judgments using caring as the justification for such statements.

If a strong definition of caring is possible and necessary, the issue then becomes, where to begin the inquiry. *Caring* is a vague and ambiguous concept requiring clarification. A vague term is usually one referring to a quality or property that is present in varying degrees, such as large, small, long and short. No rule in the English language specifies exactly how much of such a quality a thing must have in order for the term to apply. A term is ambiguous if it can receive more than one meaning. A term may be vague without being ambiguous, and it may be ambiguous without being vague. It is my hope that an analysis of the concept will dispel the vagueness and ambiguity.

Analysis of the concept of caring will proceed in three steps. First I propose to review the caring slogans in nursing literature to show the muddle and emphasize the importance of clarifying the term. Secondly, an analysis of caring in normal usage will establish the conditions necessary and sufficient to say, "X is caring for X," or in other words, given conditions 1. . .n, caring is identified. The third step involves further refinement of the conditions to strengthen the argument for this set of action categories (conditions) as justifying any instance of caring.

After the analysis, the next step involves the use of the Kerr-Soltis model of competency[21] as applied to the action categories (conditions) of caring. The question of degrees of competence in caring has strong implications for evaluation of student performance as the educator asks, "What makes S more able to care for X than for T to care for X? Can T be taught to care for X?"

Method to Study Caring

Insofar as philosophy is analytic, it primarily concerns the clarification of concepts and their relations. According to Scheffler, the basic significance of philosophical activity is "rational reflection, critical analysis of arguments and assumptions, and systematic clarification of fundamental ideas."[22]

Because philosophy is an analysis of language rather than fact, techniques of analysis are developed that help answer questions of concept rather than questions of fact or value. Scheffler identified five such techniques: 1) *structural analysis* begins by noting the logical structure of the argument under examination and then fills in omitted steps and likely assumptions; 2) *rational reconstruction* tries to render explicit the rules and special standards governing the valid inferences in given domains; 3) *semantic analysis* focuses on the typical uses of terms or concepts in ordinary language; 4) *explicative analysis* attempts to refine and explain current concepts systematically so as to render them unambiguous, precise, and theoretically adequate; and 5) *contextual analysis* stresses the dependence of concepts upon the practical contexts in which they are used by examining the function of the terms within specific situations, as well as the criteria such situations specify for their correct application.[8]

Although these methods are only ideal types and not self-sufficient tools, they demonstrate analytical philosophy's emphasis on clarity, logic, and reasoning. Scheffler identified the philosopher's task as "not striving to develop a scientific theory of languages, but rather to clarify, improve, or systematize the languages, in which we express our scientific theories, our common-sense beliefs, our judgments, inferences, evaluation, and convictions."[22]

In this study on the concept of caring, I will attempt to utilize semantic analysis in focusing on the typical uses of the term in ordinary language, explicative analysis to refine the term, and if possible, make it theoretically adequate by exploring the justifying reasons for accepting certain statements about caring as true.

Concept analysis attempts to pin down general or abstract ideas in order to bring clear conditions that must be met if a particular concept is to be strictly applicable, and thus theoretically adequate.[23] One way to identify the conditions for caring would be to watch someone engaged in such activity; then a list of actions could serve as the standard or criteria for a stipulated definition of caring. This sort of definition would be theoretical in the weak sense, for it would be no more than an arbitrary list of behaviors the observer considered to be caring. Two research studies of the caring process of nursing stipulated definitions of caring that were ambiguous and vague. Both researchers admitted that the conclusions of the studies were not as fruitful as they has initially hypothesized—to identify caring behaviors of the nurse with patient as positive factors in the relationship.[24]

To develop a description of caring in the strongest theoretical sense, one needs not only to observe actions, but also to ask questions about why X is being done, and why X is being done in a particular manner. Such questions are necessary, for practical activities nearly always improve an exercise of judgment based upon knowledge appropriate for that particular activity.[4] In its stronger sense, then, a theoretical description indicates not only what counts as caring, but also what noncaring is. It also identifies reasons, or justifies the acceptance of that particular description as theoretically adequate.[6]

A theoretically adequate description, according to Kerr and Soltis, implies that the description is general enough to cover all cases or instances of the concept and specific enough to distinguish between any two cases of the concept.[21] With the discussion of an adequate theoretical description and the weak and strong sense of that description, the reader might be led into thinking that analysis and theory are one and the same. That is not true. A theory of caring would attempt to put together a series of statements that would help to explain or predict certain empirical phenomena which one recognized as caring. The type of explanation a theory contributes to is an empirical explanation. The explaining statements are considered synthetic or *a posteriori,* in which the truth of the statement is dependent upon experiential evidence.[19]

Analysis, however, is a conceptual rather than an empirical undertaking. It involves the investigation of the term, its logic, its meaning, or its use. Analytic statements are *a priori,* which means that the truth of the statement can only be known by analysis of its structure, without dependence upon experiential evidence.[19] The analyst deals with concepts at the second level of abstraction, rather than at a behavioral level. This level is "metatheory," in which the analyst thinks about what is being thought rather than about what is being done.[25]

The questions being asked in this analysis initially have to do with the ordinary usage of the term *caring.* Normal or ordinary usage refers to the way in which a word or expression is regularly used as opposed to nonstandard uses such as metaphysical, hyperbolical, poetical, extended or deliberately restricted.[26] Instead of claiming to be giving the correct use of caring, rather, I will be looking at the employment of the term in normal usage to answer such questions as, "Why does one use the term caring in this situation and not in that?" The point of asking such questions is that the concept of caring is both vague and ambiguous, and to explicate any kind of extended definition one must first consider some instances of the concept or some cases in which the word is used to identify those uses that are nearer to the meaning of the concept than others.[27]

Having distinguished between the primary or central uses of the concept from the borderline uses, I will proceed to analyze the concept itself by a method taught by Kerr and Soltis[21] which entails setting up conditions of caring and running those conditions through a necessity/sufficiency test. When setting up the conditions for caring, I will engage in inferential reasoning that says, "If such-and-such, then so-and-so," or "if A, then B."

In any conditional statement, the first statement is the antecedent (if A) and the second statement the consequent (then B). The conditional statement that states "if A, then B" asserts a relation between two statements, the antecedent and the consequent. Any statement of this form asserts that the antecedent is the sufficient condition for the consequent, and that the consequent is a necessary condition for the antecedent. Sufficient conditions are associated with the antecedent; necessary conditions are associated with the consequent. The possibility of discovering both necessary and sufficient conditions is important for the truth of the inference.[19]

If a set of logically necessary and sufficient conditions for caring can be identified, then a definition in the strongest possible sense (theoretically adequate) has been explicated.

Having identified the necessary and sufficient conditions to speak of caring, the next step will be to generate from those conditions, a theoretically adequate description of caring. To be considered adequate, the proposed description will have to be justified as both theoretically and conceptually adequate. That is, the description meets normal usage and logical rules essential for a concept, and the generality and specificity rules which are essential for a theoretical description.

The description of caring derived from the identified caring condition will be based on consideration of caring as a purposive, intentional, human action rather than behavior. Kaplan discussed explanation in the behavioral sciences and distinguished between two senses of the statement, "What people do." The *what* may be considered as a set of acts or as a set of actions. A set of acts (behavioral description) entails biophysical operations, movements, or events. A set of actions are the acts in the perspectives of the actors, expressing certain attitudes and expectations and thereby having social and psychological significance or *act meaning*.[28]

What is most significant about this distinction for the purpose of this study is that action language takes into account intentions and purposes. Judgment of nuring actions as competent or incompetent caring must be made with reference to the nurse's intentions, purposes, and related considerations.

From an action description of caring, competencies that go beyond the mere description of discrete skills or performances will be identified. In other words, the caring competencies will be developed from a theoretical description of caring that was generated from caring conditions identified as necessary and sufficient to speak of anyone (S) caring for another (X). The adequacy with which competency in caring can be described will be directly related to the strength of the action description or analysis of the concept itself.

References

1. Nightingale F: Notes on Nursing. Philadelphia, JB Lippincott, 1946.
2. Buber M: I and Thou, translated by Walter Kaufman. New York, Charles Scribner's Sons, 1970.
3. Erikson EH: Childhood and Society, 2nd ed. New York, WW Norton, 1963.

4. Jourard S: The Transparent Self, revised ed. New York, D VanNostrand Co, 1971.
5. Rogers C: On Becoming A Person. Boston, Houghton-Mifflin Co, 1961.
6. Mayeroff M: On Caring. New York, Harper and Row, 1971.
7. Orlando IJ: The Dynamic Nurse-Patient Relationship. New York, GP Putnam and Sons, 1952.
8. Peplau H: Interpersonal Relations In Nursing. New York, Putnam and Sons, 1952.
9. Travelbee J: Interpersonal Aspects of Nursing. Philadelphia, FA Davis, 1966.
10. Henderson V: The Nature of Nursing. AJN, August, 1963, pp 62-68.
11. American Nurses Association: Educational Preparation for Nurse Practitioner and Assistants to Nurses. New York, 1965.
12. Brunner LS, Suddarth DS: Textbook of Medical-Surgical Nursing, 3rd ed. Philadelphia, JB lippincott Co, 1975.
13. Working Philosophy of Nursing. Paper presented to the Nursing Faculty, University of Washington School of Nursing, November 17, 1970.
14. Maxwell M: The Many Sources of Nursing Knowledge. Communicating Nursing Research, WICHE, November, 1972, pp 1-8.
15. Scheffler I: The Language of Education. IL, Charles Thomas, 1971.
16. Salmon WC: Logic, 2nd ed. NJ, Prentice-Hall, 1973.
17. Feigal H: On the Meaning and the Limit of Justification. In Black M (ed): Philosophical Analysis. NJ, Prentice-Hall, 1963.
18. Austin J: How To Do Things With Words. MS, Harvard University Press, 1962.
19. Green TF: The Activities of Teaching. New York, McGraw-Hill Co, 1971.
20. Gorovitz S et al: Philosophical Analysis. 2nd ed. New York, Random House, 1963.
21. Kerr D, Soltis JF: Locating Teacher Competency. Educational Theory, Vol 4, 1 (Winter): 3-16, 1974.
22. Scheffler I: Philosophy and Education. Boston, Allyn and Bacon, 1958.
23. Soltis J: An Introduction to the Analysis of Educational Cencepts. MA, Addison-Wesley Publishing Co, 1968.
24. Bush J: A Study of Surgical Patient's Perception of Selected Dimensions of Nurse-Patient Relationships and Narcotic Analgesic Intake. Thesis, University of Washington, 1973.
25. Peters RS: Ethics and Education. London, Oxford University Press, 1966.
26. Kneller G: Logic and Language of Education. New York, Wiley and Sons, 1965.
27. Wilson J: Thinking With Concepts. MA, Cambridge University Press, 1963.
28. Kaplan A: The Conduct of Inquiry. San Francisco, Chandler Publishing Co, 1964.

A Philosophical Analysis of Caring Within Nursing

Marilyn A. Ray, R.N., M.S.N.

3

Introduction and Purpose

The development and advancement of nursing knowledge among nurse educators and researchers is beginning to occur with critiques of existing theories and the discovery of the underlying epistemological basis of nursing. Contemporary nursing reflects scientific values by nature of its research, education, and practice. Nursing has been greatly influenced by theoretical developments in psychology, biology, sociology, and more recently, anthropology. Emphasis has been placed upon quantification methods to measure and validate hypothetical and theoretical statements. Indeed, much attention has been given to scientific analysis. Has this method helped to identify an underlying general thesis for nursing? Or has this method served to adopt and adapt theories or concepts from the human and behavioral sciences? I believe that theories utilized from other disciplines have not sufficiently contributed to nursing's way of formulating its essential knowledge base. Silva[1] contends that in order to study the structure of nursing knowledge, now is the time to question the scientific approach. The construct of *caring*, investigated by Leininger[2,3] along with a few other nurse scholars, hold that caring is the essence of nursing and must be studied for its meaning and value.

One way to examine the constitution of care or caring is by philosophical analysis. Philosophy, though not a science, concerns itself with science in a certain way. It is described as the science of first principles, ie, those related to meaningfulness and understanding. Metaphysics, a branch of philosophy, addresses the question: "How must the world be if it is to be intelligibly described?" Thus, to incorporate metaphysics as a means of describing meaningfulness and understanding of care or caring within nursing is to be concerned with the "whys of nursing life." Metaphysics begins with things which are believed in, but not proved.

The purpose of this paper is to develop a conceptual analysis about caring from several sources as the central philosophical belief of nursing. This analysis will aim at locating the human content and scope of caring by use of historical and contemporary sources of information and philosophies about human encounters. The final portion of the paper will focus on the formulation of a conceptual schema through philosophical analyses. This I believe will contribute to knowledge of the meaning and understanding of care as an epistemological base of nursing. This philosophical meaning of care can be made specific to nurses' responsibilities.

The History of Caring in Nursing

Dock and Nutting,[4,5] historians of nursing, called nursing the oldest of occupations for women. Their historical account juxtaposed nursing to motherhood and maternal care. They posited that the principal component in human survival is care which has been transmitted chiefly by the hands and toil of the female in interaction with her offspring. Care is evident or alluded to in the care of animals (especially by descriptions of maternal behaviors), in prehistorical records through speculation about fossil remains and in the recorded history largely through descriptions of maternal behaviors in various world cultures. Care can be identified with the concerns of many religious women engaged in humanistic services to the poor, sick, and helpless.

Nightingale,[6,7] called the "mother of modern nursing," emphasized nursing as health oriented, ie, nursing was to put people in the best condition for Nature to restore or preserve health and to prevent or cure disease or injury. She believed that the nurse must have simplicity and a single eye to the patient's good. Nightingale also emphasized that nursing was usually performed by women under scientific heads (physicians and surgeons) who prescribed treatments for the sick to be carried out by nurses. She also looked upon nursing as involving a form of manual labor, evolving from the traditional role of women, regardless of the motivation which prompted the service. For example, along with the care of the sick, dying, and injured, housekeeping activities in the form of cleaning, scrubbing, doing laundry, managing the kitchen, and cooking were perceived to be in the realm of nursing by Nightingale.

Nightingale,[6,7] pointed to nursing as the art of charity—"God's work"—as she expressed it. A good nurse, according to Nightingale, was of the highest class of character (in earlier times in England, women selected for nursing came from the lower classes) and was to be the Sermon on the Mount in herself, ie, honest, truthful, trustworthy, hopeful, orderly, and thinking of others rather than of herself. A nurse was to be tender, cheerful, kind, patient, and ingenious. In short, a nurse was to be *good* and *loving*.

Caring Perspectives in Current Nursing Literature

Leininger[2] states that nursing is derived from the concept of nurturance which includes ideas of caring, growth, and support. She also holds that caring is the dominant intellectual, theoretical, heuristic, and central practice focus of nursing, and no other profession is so totally concerned with caring behaviors, caring processes, and caring relationships than nursing. To support this claim, Leininger developed a classification of ethnocaring constructs from her ethnoscientific research of approximately 30 cultures. Some of these concepts discovered are comfort measures, support measures, compassion, empathy, nurturance, surveillance, touching, health instructive acts, and others.

Bevis[8] developed a conceptual framework delineating phases of caring from a grounded theory approach. Bevis believes that the purpose of caring is intimately joined with some health forms of love. Caring impels one to create an environment for loved ones that enables them to fulfill themselves. Therefore, the purpose of caring is growth and mutual self-actualization.

Watson[9] defined the caring process as encompassing factors that help the person attain (or maintain) health or die a peaceful death. The factors which form the structure for understanding nursing as the science of caring establish a means for promoting positive health changes—for example, the formation of humanistic/altruistic systems of values, the instillation of faith and hope, the cultivation of mutual sensitivity, the development of a helping/trusting relationship and a supportive environment, assistance with the gratification of human needs, the promotion of interpersonal teaching and learning, and the use of problem solving techniques for decision-making.

Paterson and Zderad, authors of *Humanistic Nursing,*[10] identified nursing behavior in terms of an existential view of man* as "in process"—becoming or moving toward self-actualization. Their inner perspective model is represented by what Buber calls the "I-Thou" dialogical relationship. The meaning of humanistic nursing is found in the human act itself. The authors explained that the elements of this humanistic framework include incarnate men (patient and nurse) meeting (being and becoming) in a goal-directed (nurturing wellbeing and more-being), intersubjective transaction (being with and doing with) occurring in time and space (as measured and lived by patient and nurse) in a world of men and things. When nursing is genuinely humanistic, nursing is an expression, a living out of the nurse's authentic commitment. Patterson and Zderad speak of nursing as an existential engagement directed toward nurturing human potential.

From these expressed or implied accounts of caring and nursing, a recurrent theme is that caring refers to growth or mutual self-actualization. To understand the growth process in a caring relationship, Mayeroff[11] characterizes the concept in the following way:

> To help another person grow is at least to help him to care for something or someone apart from himself, and it involves encouraging and assisting him to find and create areas of his own in which he is able to care. Also, it is to help that

---

**No distinction is made with respect to gender in this paper.*

other person to come to care for himself, and by becoming responsive to his own need to care to become responsible for his own life.

From early historical perspectives where caring centered in the mother-child relationship to the evolution of caring in nursing, the notion of growth or nurturing the wellbeing of another is a central focus of nursing. But is this belief upheld in practice situations, or in most educational institutions where nursing knowledge is disseminated, or in research where caring is often subjected to methods of positivistic science? Recent data suggest that in our over-bureaucratized health care system all efforts toward creating persons who are responsible for their own lives in matters of health are diminished. What has happened to the caring ideology in nursing?

The Recent Situation in Nursing Within North American Cultures

Nursing care takes place primarily within institutional settings like hospitals or nursing homes, and a portion of professional nursing takes place within the community health sector. Nursing in hospitals is becoming increasingly technological and bureaucratic. Community health nursing is becoming increasingly managerial and supervisory. A dilemma for nursing, relative to its central focus as a direct caring profession, has thus occurred.

Technical-scientific advances and the competition for physician services within hospital bureaucracies have led to the production and promulgation of the "curing syndrome", and to an adoption of the medical symptomatic cure model of surgery and/or medication within hospitals.[12] In order to satisfy the need to meet technological demands, care (both individual and collective) has been receiving less and less emphasis. Given the relative powerlessness of nurses *vis-a-vis* physicians and administrators and the problem of insurance company control over health care expenditures, nursing has been unable to sustain its caring ideology.

In the public health domain, the possibility for promoting and re-emphasizing a caring ideology with home health situations has fallen victim to the role and value system of nurses as managers administering only indirect care. Those nurses in direct care are named "therapeutic" nurses and are often relegated to the low status ranks within the professional nursing hierarchy.

Of importance to nursing are the changing sex roles in the Western world. Motherhood, male roles, and the subservient position of women have all come under scrutiny in recent years. Changes in the work ideology for women have produced conflict between the home and the marketplace. Bronfenbrenner,[13] a social scientist in child care research, elaborated on the "empty home" symbol in American culture as the symbol of "nobody caring."

Male sex roles are changing slowly. Nurturant male behavior has not been encouraged, and those males who enter the nursing profession are often condemned by the larger society as being odd, or gay. But males who enter and remain in nursing generally move quickly to administrative positions, health care specialty areas such as anesthesiology or psychiatry, and/or physician-linked roles such as the physician assistant. Hence, their male identification is closely linked to physician or bureaucratic-managerial interests, freeing them from a close association with the female-nurturant roles.

Institutions and community health systems appear to be incongruent with professional caring. Given the structural value system, economic competition, and the entrenchment of health care settings with the medical model of diagnosis, treatment, and ultimately cure, caring values are submerged. These values lead to conflicts within nursing. On the one hand, nursing claims to have a caring ideology and a humanistic approach. On the other hand, actual conduct usually meets the demands of a bureaucratic value system, the world of physician-centered interests and technological values, and now the self-interests of nurses themselves.[12] The consequences, in short, are the widening disparity between belief and action, and confusion and despair within the professional ranks.

This dilemma, resulting from *carers* being forced by circumstances *away from the caring* to which they are pledged, puts patient/clients in the vulnerable position of receiving poor or little care, which neither promotes nor enhances growth in wellbeing or wellness. For example, nurses who unquestionably follow a medical-symptomatic cure model, especially relative to aged patients, contribute to alterations in the quality of life; that is, lives dominated by excessive medication, unnecessary surgeries, repeated hospitalizations, and dependence upon the cold technological health care system of today.

Thus, the caring behavior of nursing is threatened. Preservation of human and humane caring—human-to-human interaction—is an issue to which nurses must pay close attention. Today's challenge is the reaffirmation of the *human* scope of care by showing how the caring component must be re-established as central to nursing. The following section of this essay will examine caring, using philosophical perspectives in an attempt to rediscover and understand the human content of caring behavior in nursing.

What Caring Involves

To address the notion of caring from philosophical perspectives, I will present aspects of the philosophies of Marcel and Buber, and some material will illuminate the work of humanistic nursing by Paterson and Zderad.[10] To emphasize the humanistic element of nursing, historical references to Nightingale's beliefs about nursing and contemporary sources of caring knowledge from interviews with children and women will be used. The relationship of caring to loving becomes self-evident during this discourse. To begin, I will use the distinctions drawn by Marcel between problem and mystery to facilitate an understanding of the concept of *co-presense* or the active participation of nurse with patient/client in professional nursing situations.[14]

Marcel characterized the great perennial questions of human life as mysteries involving the questioner himself, distinguishing them from ordinary problems upon which it is possible to take a more detached, objective point of view. Marcel affirmed that questions affecting human life represented in terms of mystery find the questioner involved in the data of the question; that is, rather than being outside the data, the questioner is concerned with, touched or affected by, and included in the data of the question.[14] As examples, the meaning of hope or fidelity, the realities of an I-thou encounter, of presence, and of hope are not confronted as problems to be solved but lived, greeted, or welcomed. The subject-object dichotomy dissolves and is transcended. Thus, the structure of mystery with its co-presence of subject-object, its fusion of questioner and reality in question is properly that of an encounter implying an active subject's presence to the presence of an encountered reality.[15] The illumination of the concept of mystery (the mystery of co-presence) is brought into focus by the process of reflection, and Marcel's explication characterizes its final distinctive trait as permanence. That is, rather than objectifying data as in the the problem-solving approach—the usual approach in nursing—a mystery is continuously penetrated and clarified while still being retained, which is indicative of open-endedness, and suggestive of new beginnings, or of the idea of growing and becoming.[15]

To support Marcel's view, Buber exemplified the notion of intersubjective relationships or co-presence by his philosophical anthropology. According to Friedman, Buber's philosophy points at the "sphere of between" which is common to both. Buber called the unfolding of this sphere the dialogical. The meaning of the dialogue is found in neither one nor the other of the partners, nor in both taken together, but in their interchange. It is a question of the authenticity of what is between men, without which there can be no authentic human existence.[16]

Buber wrote that dialogue can be either spoken or silent. The essential element is "seeing the other", or "experiencing the other side". What is meant by this notion is to feel an event from the side of the person one meets as well as from one's own side. It is not to be confused with empathy, however, which means transposing one's self into the dynamic structure of the object—to the exclusion of one's own concreteness. Instead, experiencing the other side is the extension of one's own concreteness, the fulfillment of the actual situation of life, the complete presence of the reality in which one participates. Experiencing the other side is the essence of all genuine love.[16]

The ideas of mystery, presence, and dialogue, as developed by Marcel and Buber, yield a foundational account of caring in general, and therefore of nursing care as a particular application. The following data, gathered in discussions with groups of women and children, and drawing from Nightingale's writings, may assist in the transition from the abstract philosophical characterization to a more concrete account of nursing care.

Two 11 year old boys were asked what they thought care was. One boy stated, "Care is how people care for you—your mother or your father." The other boy remarked, "Remember what our teacher said. You can't define a term with the same term." The boy who spoke first began again by exclaiming, "Well, it's like CARE—the people who take care of foster children." He continued, "It is love—like parents—they care for you, give you things, help you."

A group of women were asked by the author to present their ideas about care. The following are their ideas as they were expressed in writing:

> Caring is sharing the gifts that God has given to us.
>
> Care is to reach out in love with love. It is going beyond what is required. It is giving and not wanting anything in return. It is just love.
>
> Care is the willingness to give of time, energy, love, prayer, or whatever is needed at what time it is needed—even when one doesn't feel like giving, or when the time is inconvenient.
>
> Caring means the willingness to put another person and his/her needs before one's own.
>
> Care and caring are being for others.
>
> Care is when your concern for another comes before your concern for yourself.
>
> Caring means giving, not of money, or material things, but of your total self, total being—stepping into the other's shoes, understanding, so that you can *care* and meet their needs.
>
> Caring is to listen, to be present or available to another even when the time is inconvenient. It is to touch, to reach out to others, to smile, to encourage, to praise, and to give of one's self without reservation.
>
> Care is to welcome by a smile or a word or a presence. It is to listen but not only for receiving everything from the other. It is not to feel superior because we listen, but to share with him and to be open and, if possible, without *a priori*. It is to be simple and "poor" in our relations, and to permit the other to be comfortable—to be himself.

From these contemporary sources, it is evident that caring is perceived as involving a process of co-presence, giving, receiving, communication, and in essence loving in the sense that Marcel[17] conveyed; that is, oblative love or other-directedness.

In a recent study conducted by Gardner and her co-worker, Wheeler, (unpublished data, 1979) they reported that two concepts, *love* and *nearness with love,* were important phrases rated by staff nurses in relation to the concept of support, having factor analytic Eigen value loadings of .85 and .83 respectively (Eigen value 1.0).

Nightingale[7] epitomized nurses as loving by representing nursing behavior as the ultimate of Christian love. Nightingale, presupposing a Christian community of nurses, viewed nurses as incarnations of the Sermon on the Mount and the Beatitudes. The following is a text of Christ's words as reported in Matthew 5:1-12:

> Blest are the poor in Spirit; the reign of God is theirs.
>
> Blest too are the sorrowing; they shall be consoled.
>
> Blest are the lowly; they shall inherit the land.
>
> Blest are they who hunger and thirst for holiness; they shall have their fill.
>
> Blest are they who show mercy; mercy shall be theirs.
>
> Blest are the single hearted; for they shall see God.
>
> Blest too are the peace-makers; they shall be called the sons of God.
>
> Blest are those persecuted for holiness sake; the reign of God is theirs.
>
> Blest are you when they insult you and persecute you and utter every kind of slander against you because of me.
>
> Be glad and rejoice, for your reward is great in heaven; they persecuted the prophets before you in the very same way.

Though concern is expressed between God and the individual, the social implications of the Sermon on the Mount are evident. Nightingale believed nurses were to be of the highest moral character and equated them with the Beatitudes, ie, religious happiness. Dedication to the ideals of giving, helping, compassion, loyalty, constancy, and freedom from material gain were to be socially practiced in the care of the sick. In essence, the concept of nursing conceived and practiced by Nightingale was apparently in the image of God as all-loving, and all-good. Nightingale exemplified these ideals, too, in her work among the war victims of the Crimea in the mid-nineteenth century. She concluded with the following passage in her famous book *Notes on Nursing:*

> ...go your way straight to God's work, in simplicity and singleness of heart.[6]

Thus, a conceptual analysis of caring from different perspectives is suggestive of a form of loving (oblative or other-directed love) where co-presence in human encounter is a mystery rather than a problem to be solved, and where growth is fostered through effective dialogue. The meaning of caring as loving may be viewed as complex, but Teilhard de Chardin spoke of the universality of love:[18]

> Love is the most universal, the most tremendous, and the most mysterious of cosmic forces...It is the primal and universal psychic energy.

Furthermore, Teilhard de Chardin stated that socially, in science, business, and public affairs, men pretend not to know love, though under the surface it is everywhere. These ideas can be extended to institutions where *care* is provided and where nurses may pretend not to know love (care). Perhaps, because caring is such an overwhelming responsibility, high demands placed upon nurses may speak to the impossible, thus rendering our historical and contemporary ideologies invalid in today's cultural context. However, if we adopt the view that a reaffirmation of the human content and scope of caring within nursing must be re-established, then the task of examining and altering the current culture of nursing must be confronted.

Caring and Nursing Today

Blanshard states:[19]

> Philosophy is to understand; to understand is to explain; and to explain is to place things in a context that reveals them as necessary. Such explanation is genuine discovery.

The following is a visual and proposed representation of the concepts discovered by a metaphysical analysis of caring representing co-presence and love as nursing:

Conceptual Scheme of Caring Representing Co-Presence and Love as the Essential Nature of Nursing*

Co-Presence

Authenticity
Availability
Attendance
Communication
- **Interest**
- **Acceptance**
- **Touch**
- **Empathy**

Oblative Love ↕ **Giving and Receiving**

Engaging in philosophical analysis of caring as the heart of the normative context of nursing leads us to a heightened awareness of our overwhelming responsibility if a caring process is to be central to professional behavior. The following portion of this essay will elucidate how the theoretical results of the analysis can be made specific to nurses' responsibilities, how practical results of the responsibilities can be made specific to the work activities of nurses, and finally, how benefits and improvements can be gained from adopting this philosophical view.

The theoretical results of a philosophical analysis should be introduced to nursing faculty, nurses, and student nurses by means of education, ie, basic and graduate nursing education and continuing education programs, and by means of the professional literature. Philosophy is equally as important as science! One must be cognizant, however, that a pervasive awareness of *caring* in nursing cannot be achieved merely through knowledge of philosophical analysis and/or scientific explanations, but must be realized and felt in one's own life. Bronfenbrenner[13] believed that caring behavior may have to be taught since, in American society, within their own homes children are less and less exposed to role models expressing care. Thus, a specific type of education, an analysis of the nurse's own experiences of care, will reveal the extent to which her/his caring for others may be accomplished. Bevis' account[8] of phases of caring may assist in facilitating this goal.

**Acknowledgment is given to Gardner for her encouragement, help, and research data on support behaviors in the development of a model of caring.*

A normative theoretical position on care can facilitate the much needed continuation of philosophical inquiry and empirical research into the phenomenon of care itself. Nurses are adopting a technological-cure bureaucratic model for practice.[12] Research on caring behaviors is needed as expressed by adopting such a model. How is technology used? Is it a medium of care, or does it become an end in itself with respect to nurse-patient interaction? Also, the cure model of surgery and medication, although not new to nurses, must receive greater emphasis. Research into these areas of conflict will allow for increased understanding and explanation of the roles of physicians and medicine in relation to nurses and nursing. In relation to the bureaucratic model, nursing research is imperative for determining the extent to which the influences of structural characteristics and bureaucratic values of institutions affect the care behavior of nurses.[20]

Will the results of research about care suggest a realignment of the care ideology of nurses to the realities of practice? How well is our caring ideology manifested in today's nursing? Do nurses want to care, and do patients want to receive care?

Another area for explication is how the practical results of an analysis of care can be made specific to the work activities of nurses. Education again can be the prime source of motivation. However, in the arena of practice, education of nurses is not sufficient by itself. Changes in institutions (hospitals and community organizations) are contingent upon the following factors: an awareness of bureaucratic and physician values and interests, economic considerations, the physician and nurse hierarchies, client rights in home health care, and technology and total schema of health/cure/care provisioning. Can systems be changed to include humane caring?

Still another important area of nursing practice is the reward system for nurses. Nurses, for the most part, have been rewarded only for supporting the bureaucratic management system, for following physician orders, and improving their technical skills. Additional caring rendered to patients generally does not reap benefits. Lalonde[21] exclaimed that health professionals still tend to regard the human body as a biological machine which can be kept running by removing or replacing defective parts or by clearing clogged lines. At best, this view is only a partial perspective on the management of health and illness. As Lalonde argued, the values of the health care system will have to be changed so that care will be raised to the same level of importance as cure. Are nurses capable of assuming responsibility for putting caring values into practice? Can care become a marketable commodity? If so, how much should it be worth?

By developing authentic caring relationships in work situations, nurses can experience intrinsic rewards such as increased self-esteem, job satisfaction, motivation, and joy in giving and receiving. Mayeroff[11] wrote that besides the other's need for me if he is to grow, I need the other to care for, if I am to be myself. He also emphasized that caring is not always agreeable; it is sometimes frustrating, and rarely easy. Therefore, in the process of caring there is both pain and joy; but caring aids in the discovery and creation of the meaning of life both within the professional nursing context and within one's own personal life.

Patients will benefit by recognizing that caring is actually taking place. Through caring, patients should experience a special type of *love* to assist them in the restoration or maintenance of health or to provide the environment necessary for a peaceful death. Though physicians do not overwhelmingly respond positively to suggestions from nurses, physicians could experience increased benefits in terms of caring by witnessing more rapid recovery rates of patients with less tendency for repeated admissions to hospitals.[22] Also, physicians could gain greater intrinsic rewards by understanding their role as *physician-carers* rather than purely curers, and by beginning to understand the extent to which care by nurses is intricately woven into the recovery process of patients. Physicians can learn, therefore, that the wellbeing of patients is not their exclusive domain.

By increasing *caring,* institutions could benefit by establishing a reordering of their value systems in the direction of greater overall societal benefit. If institutions adopted caring as a primary source of operational motivation, there could be far-reaching effects transmitted to insurance companies, other institutions that form the network of interchange with hospitals such as supply and pharmaceutical houses, and the society which supports the hospitals. An increased awareness of the value of caring could revolutionize society at large. Moreover, nurses who believe they possess the potential to help other people grow must assume that responsibility by advancing their caring beliefs so that the process touches, affects, and changes lives. Ultimately, caring must be the goal to reverse the noncaring behaviors in Western culture to which the social scientist Bronfenbrenner[13] has made reference. The responsibility of practicing a caring ideology for nurses is great, but the responsibility for not caring is even greater.

References

1. Silva MC: Philosophy, Science, Theory: Interrelationships and Implications for Nursing Research. Image, Vol 9, 3:59-63, 1977.
2. Leininger M: The Phenomenon of Caring—Caring: The Essence and Central Focus of Nursing. American Nurses' Foundation, March:2, 14, 1977.
3. Leininger M: Transcultural Nursing: Concepts, Theories and Practices. New York, John Wiley & Sons, 1978, pp 33, 39.
4. Dock L, Stewart IM: A Short History of Nursing. New York, GP Putnam's Sons, 1920.
5. Nutting MA, Dock L: A History of Nursing. Vol I. New York, GP Putnam and Sons, 1935.
6. Nightingale F: Notes on Nursing. New York, D Appleton and Co, 1860, pp 135-136.
7. Seymer LR: Selected Writings of Florence Nightingale. New York, The MacMillan Company, 1954, p 351.
8. Bevis EO: Conceptual Framework: The Knowledge Component. In Curriculum Building in Nursing: A Process, 2nd ed. St. Louis, MO, CV Mosby & Co, 1978, pp 110-122.
9. Watson J: Nursing: The Philosophy and Science of Caring. Boston, Little, Brown and Company, 1979, pp 7-10.
10. Patterson J, Zderad L: Humanistic Nursing. New York, John Wiley & Sons, 1976, pp 16, 23.

11. Mayeroff, M: On Caring. New York, Harper & Row, publishers, 1971, pp 11, 224-52.
12. Ray MA: An Applied Anthropological Study of Role Behavior Within the Profession of Nursing Within the Complex Institution of the Hospital. Thesis, McMaster University, Hamilton, Ontario, Canada, 1978.
13. Bronfenbrenner U: Nobody Home: The Erosion of the American Family. Psychology Today, Vol 10, 12:4-47, 1977.
14. Marcel G: The Philosophy of Existence. New York, Philosophical Library, 1949.
15. Hanley K, Monan JH: A Prelude to Metaphysics. Englewood Cliffs, NJ, Prentice-Hall, Inc, 1967, pp 84-86.
16. Friedman, M: Martin Buber: The Life of Dialogue. Chicago, The University of Chicago Press, 1976, pp 85-88.
17. Marcel G: Presence and Immortality. Pittsburgh, Duquesne University Press, 1967, p 235.
18. Teilhard de Chardin. On Love. New York, Harper & Row Publishers, 1967, pp 7-8.
19. Blanshard B: The Philosophy of Analysis. In Lewis, HO (ed): Clarity Is Not Enough. New York, Humanities Press Inc, 1969, p 76.
20. Ashley J: Hospitals, Paternalism, and the Role of the Nurse. New York, Teachers' College Press, 1976.
21. Lalonde M: A New Perspective on the Health of Canadians. Ottawa, Ontario, Government of Canada, 1974, pp 24, 41.
22. Wolfer J, Visintainer M: Pediatric Surgical Patients' and Parents' Stress and Response and Adjustment. Nursing Research. Vol 24, 4:244-255, 1975.

An Application of the Structural-Functional Method to the Phenomenon of Caring

Joyceen S. Boyle, R.N., M.P.H.

4

Introduction

There is a crucial need for nurse theorists to begin to develop theories of nursing. This urgency has increased since professional nursing has begun to make its way among other university-based disciplines. Evans-Pritchard[1] observed that a subject of scholarship can hardly be said to have autonomy before it is taught in the universities. In this sense, professional nursing is a new subject. As the focus of the health care delivery system swings toward promotion and maintenance of health and away from the curing of illness, nursing needs to define and clarify the contribution that nursing care makes to the preservation and improvement of various conditions of human life.

Jacox[2] observed that a practice is only as good as the knowledge on which it is based. Unfortunately, efforts to develop and test knowledge for nursing practice have not matched the enthusiasm for improving that practice. It is distressing to encounter professional nurses who cannot explain what nursing is and who believe that, at best, nursing consists of willy-nilly bits and pieces of other disciplines that are somehow "changed" into nursing by practical application. A general theory of nursing is also required to give scope and direction to the search being conducted under the guise of nursing research. The publishing of more and more about less and less is an acceptable quest only if it does not lead to neglect or obfuscation of the more fundamental issues. It may be possible to defend the so-called nursing mini-theories in relation to research interest, the idea being that work can proceed on an eclectic, piecemeal basis in anticipation that someday all of the pieces of the puzzle will fit together and we will then have general theories of nursing. However, Harris[3] warned that such electicism abounds with hidden dangers. He pointed out that in practice it is often little more than a euphemism for confusion, the muddled acceptance of contradictory theories, the bankruptcy of creative thought and the cloak of mediocrity. It bestows upon its practitioners a false sense of security and an unearned reputation for scientific acumen.

There are many nurses who genuinely believe that it is impossible to develop nursing theories. They argue that there cannot be a defined body of knowledge that belongs uniquely to nursing. This point of view is unacceptable; theories of nursing are indeed possible, and the time is ripe for their development. Generalizations about any sort of subject matter are of two kinds: the generalizations of common opinion or superficial experiences and generalizations that have been verified or demonstrated by a systematic examination of evidence afforded by precise observations systematically made. Generalizations of the latter kind are called scientific principles or laws and are the core of any theory.[4] Those who hold that there are no laws of nursing cannot hold that there are no generalizations about nursing, because they themselves hold such generalizations and even make new ones of their own.

Purpose

The purpose of this paper is to develop a theory of nursing that systematically describes and explains the caring process in nursing practice. Various concepts contributing to the caring process will be described and examined as well as their relationship to each other and to the phenomenon of caring. The ultimate goal, although it may not be possible within the scope of this paper, is to formulate generalizations about the caring phenomenon. This theory should be of interest to nurse theorists who are attempting to integrate caring phenomenon and caring behaviors into nursing theories; it is anticipated that eventually such theories will have merit for those who practice and teach professional nursing.

The method used here to develop generalizations about nursing has been utilized in British social anthropology, particularly by Radcliffe-Brown,[4] and is known as the structural-functional method. This approach was chosen because it allows one to deal only with the entity of caring, to separate the caring process into component parts, and then to systematically conceptualize caring from a structural-functional viewpoint that facilitates a description of the interrelatedness and interdependency of the component parts.

Theoretical Developments in Nursing

Ellis[5] observed that theory development relevant to the profession of nursing requires attention to the stated or implied preposition used to connect the word *theory,* or the term *theory development* to the word *nursing.* The phrase *for nursing* implies the characteristics of the theory will be relevant to that function which has to do with assisting clients to cope with health problems. This implies some sort of applied action within the practice of nursing. For many nurse theorists, this assumption determines which theories are significant. While we recognize that nursing generally does not occur apart from clients, it has been this aspect that had led to the development of theories for nursing that have focused on holistic man and the interactional process between nurse and clients. These theories give us some feeling for what man is, how he relates to his environment, and how the nurse assists him in this context. The latter emphasizes the nursing process or applied aspects of nursing, while the former deals with the theoretical aspects of holistic man.

On the other hand, Andreoli and Thompson[6] suggest that the phrase *theory of nursing* refers to the body of verifiable knowledge that will be derived from nursing practice. It consists of a synthesis, reorganization, or extension of concepts drawn from the basic and other applied sciences which in their reformulation tend to become new concepts.

Walker[7] defined nursing as "one or more persons caring for the physical and mental wellbeing of one or more persons with actual or potential health problems within a setting." She broke this definition down into subsets for further study: 1) persons providing care; 2) persons with health problems receiving care; 3) the environment where care is given, and 4) the end state—wellbeing. The emphasis is on persons, environment, and health. A crucial beginning for the development of nursing theory is an area where nursing stands uniquely at a distance from other disciplines, such as *care* itself, which is not addressed by Walker.

One legitimate purpose of a theory of nursing would be to develop theoretical perspectives about the process of caring, not about persons receiving nursing care, the environment in which nursing care is given, or the patient's responses to care. This does not in any way negate the other theoretical perspectives for nursing theories, but to be significant, a theory must be a theory *of nursing,* one that focuses primarily on the study of nursing and particularly on the process of caring. When the phenomenon of nursing can be understood and described, then predictions regarding its outcome in conjunction with a client, his environment, and health status can be stated.

Nursing is a nascent science, and nurse theorists must come to terms with how to develop and expand its knowledge base. A difference of opinion with the kind of knowledge that is being developed by nurse theorists has already been discussed, ie, that theories seem to be directed toward theories *for nursing* rather than theories *of nursing.* Nursing's embryonic stage, however, poses another interesting dilemma. How should nurse theorists proceed to develop a comprehensive and meaningful theory of nursing? If nurses believe that nursing theory is more than borrowed bits and pieces from other disciplines, then what approaches should be used to develop and expand a body of knowledge that is uniquely nursing? Does the scientific development of knowledge emerge only through developmental phases? Kuhn[8] suggests that scientific knowledge progresses by paradigms and that such progression is orderly, efficient, and logical; but he also warned that there is no shortcut or hasty road to scientific development of knowledge.

To describe the caring phenomenon in nursing, a basic approach to the development of theory must be used in the initial phases. This is the primary reason that a structural-functional methodology was chosen for this paper, although it is recognized that it does have a number of limitations. This method is a relatively static approach that freezes its subject and does not show movement or dynamics as well as other methods, such as system analysis. However, the structural-functional method does facilitate the description and interrelatedness of component parts as well as their interdependency.

Philosophy of Nursing And Clarification of Method

Many nursing theorists, such as Roy, Levine, and Rogers, have explained nursing by demonstrating its utility in maintaining health and alleviating illness. Such explanations are based on the assumption that nursing can be explained only from the point of view of the nurse's role and with no other determining factors besides the services that nurses render. Such theories only establish that society has a need for nursing care and that nursing does indeed perform a necessary service. To show how a phenomenon is useful is not to explain why it is what it is. The uses such explanations serve presuppose the specific properties characterizing nursing but do not create them. The need of society for nursing cannot give it existence, nor can it confer a specific nature upon it. It is to causes or explanations of another sort that the phenomenon of nursing owes its existence. The causes or explanations of nursing are independent of the ends it serves, so to seek an explanation of nursing, nurse theorists must critically examine the nature of nursing itself.

The structural-functional method uses the model of the biological organism as a basis for understanding social phenomena. The utilization of this model is based on the belief that social phenomena are just as real as are individual organisms and share certain similarities in that they have structural continuities and life processes which have a function important to the maintenance of that organism.[4]

Nursing and Caring

To turn now from this organic analogy to nursing, the first assumption that is tentatively made is that nursing has a social structure and a number of component parts. It is suggested that a major structural component of nursing is the phenomenon of caring. Caring is a part of nursing but is not its totality. Other major components of nursing might be counseling and curing phenomena. It is not within the scope of this paper to examine the total structure of nursing; nevertheless, other components of nursing do provide areas for further investigation. Leininger[9] points out that the discipline of nursing has traditionally been concerned with the caring needs of people, and although caring practices are of interest to other health professionals, they have not been the dominant area of focus as they are in nursing. She states that "caring is the essence of nursing and is the most central and unifying force for nursing decisions, practices, and goals. No construct could be more central, more essential, and more promising for teaching, research, and practice than ideas related to care and caring for the nurisng profession." To care for someone within the scope of professional nursing is to feel interest in and concern for the health and wellbeing of another. Mitchell[10] defined caring as that relationship that expresses the feeling of concern, regard, or respect one human being has for another. The humanness of caring was expressed by Naugle,[10] who wrote of its human dignity, its respect for life and living, for a person and not for a body. Mayeroff[11] observed that caring is more than merely interest. He felt the essence of caring is a deep regard for another, and sees caring as a basis for helping another. Caring is a crucial and vital component in nursing. In the Radcliffe-Brown sense, nurses would, through caring, provide structural continuity to nursing. Without this continuity, nursing care could not be maintained or would be incomplete.

Clients often relate episodes they have experienced in hospitals or clinics where the nursing care has been given in an impersonal and perfunctory manner. Nurses occasionally find themselves concentrating exclusively on technical skills and withdrawing from relationships which provide personal and functional care for clients. This kind of nursing lacks wholeness; its continuity has been altered—the caring component is missing.

A systematic investigation of the component of caring raises a number of problems. First is the problem of the structure of nursing itself. All the components of nursing have not been identified, and this paper will focus only on caring, which is only one aspect of the nursing structure. Therefore, caring will be described and explained as if it were a total structure. Second, what is this structure and how does it function? Again, this paper can only examine certain pieces of the puzzle but must assume that it deals with the whole. It is convenient to use the analogy between social life and organic life, but like all analogies it should be used with caution because there is a point where the analogy between organism and social phenomena breaks down. In an animal organism it is possible to observe the organic structure to some extent independent of its functioning. In other words, it is possible to make a morphology which is independent of physiology.[4] But in social life, the structural entity is an abstract representation which can be described and interpreted but cannot always be directly observed with its interdependent, interacting aspects.

The Structural Continuity of Caring

The continuity of caring as a structure is maintained by social processes consisting of the activities and interactions of nurses with patients or clients. The function of these social processes consists of the contribution they make to the structural continuity of caring. Any number of functions may contribute to the structural continuity of caring. The concept of function as a contribution is vital to this methodology. The functions of caring refer to those relations that interface the structure of caring and the various processes or parts of the system that have their roots in the application of nursing practice. The total structure of caring together with the totality of social usages or processes in which structure appears, and on which it depends for its existence, has a certain kind of unity which can be described as a functional unity. It is that condition in which all parts of the system work together with a sufficient degree of internal consistency. The stability of caring depends upon integration of its parts and the performance by these parts of particular tasks necessary for the maintenance of the form. The integration of parts and their particular tasks are the functions that maintain caring. In a structural-functional sense, these functions or contributions are the causes or explanations of caring phenomena.

For a brief review following the Radcliffe-Brown[4] conceptualization, there are three vital concepts used in the structural-functional analysis of caring: processes, function, and structure. The object of this theory is the social structure of caring and the processes or activities of caring that occur in nursing practice. The contributions that the functions fulfill arise from the processes and preserve the continuity of caring as a social structure.

Application of the Method

The concept of function as defined above constitutes a working hypothesis by which a number of problems can be formulated for investigation. No scientific inquiry is possible without a focus or formulation of such a hypothesis. This does not require the dogmatic assertion that everything about a social process has a function; it merely requires the assumption that it may have one and justifies efforts to determine what those functions may be. Since the function of a social activity is to be found by examining its effect on the social structure, a number of aspects of social process must be closely investigated and considered in relationship to one another. An essential part of the task is the investigation of the relations between social processes and how they articulate to relate in such a manner that caring can be demonstrated.

Caring is made explicitly in a system of interrelated processes between nurses and their clients, but aspects of caring are not always formally recognized by nurses. If caring is the most crucial component of nursing, then an attempt must be made to make it more explicit and to describe what is otherwise unclear.

Caring may exist on a number of analytic levels, but it is not always a creation of thought—although it is sometimes only accessible by thought rather than by observation alone. The following example and analysis attempt to describe nursing activities and a systematic framework of caring that will make the structure more understandable and consistent:

> The head nurse's first encounter with Mrs. Davidson occurred when the client was brought unexpectedly to the unit, followed by a cart stacked high with personal items, and accompanied by her husband. The unit was crowded; Mrs. Davidson was temporarily placed in the hallway. This was the last straw as far as Mr. Davidson was concerned and he expressed his frustration over his wife's situation to the head nurse.[11] Nursing activities initiated to allay the anxiety and frustration of Mr. and Mrs. Davidson were directed toward the goal of assisting Mrs. Davidson as quickly and as comfortably as possible into her own room. The

head nurse spent a few minutes with the Davidsons to explain that as soon as housekeeping personnel arrived and cleaned the room, Mrs. Davidson would be moved into it. She told them she had already made the telephone call to housekeeping and they were on their way to the unit. In the meantime, some of Mrs. Davidson's possessions were placed in an adjacent conference room and a chair was obtained for Mr. Davidson so he could sit comfortably next to his wife. The nurse who was responsible for Mrs. Davidson's care paused by the couple, introduced herself, and brought Mrs. Davidson a glass of water.

All of these nursing activities were directed toward making Mr. and Mrs. Davidson more comfortable and at ease in an unfamiliar environment. If the nurses involved in the interactions with the Davidsons were asked to explain what they were doing and why, they would undoubtedly have said that their various nursing activities were directed toward meeting identified nursing needs of the client. Their nursing care was implemented to relieve anxiety, provide reassurance that she would be placed in a room as quickly as possible, involve her husband in support of his wife, and even to administer adequate hydration, ie, the glass of water.

If these same processes are viewed within the framework of the structural-functional model, the structure of caring is symbolized and reflected in the activities, processes, and though patterns of the nursing staff. These activities mirror professionally defined relationships between nurses and their clients. Yet as indicated previously, the nurses themselves probably would speak of meeting patients' needs or of the actual nursing procedures and activities that occurred. The phenomenon of caring would probably not be mentioned, yet it is clearly present. Caring concepts guide and shape the actions of the nurses as they perform nursing activities. These activities have the function of maintaining the structure of caring. As this point, a distinction has been made between what nurses say, imagine, and conceive about themselves and their professional practice and the abstracted reality that a nursing theory requires. This is the contrast between observer-orientation and actor-orientation and is an integral part of the methodology used here. This approach is based upon the assumption that the actual participants in nursing are not always capable of an objective description of their own behavior or of a scientifically valid explanation of that behavior. The structural-functional approach attempts to clear away the rationalized appearance of things in order to penetrate into deeper levels of thought and action and to offer explanations.

With this example of nursing care, an attempt can be made to examine the nursing processes and activities and to define the contributions they make to the caring structure. All of them involve some aspect of *comfort.* Comforting is the process by which a nurse does something for clients which they cannot do for themselves, or would do for themselves if they were physically or emotionally able. Mrs. Davidson and her husband were experiencing anxiety, and the nurses responded by appropriately defined nursing activities. The resolution of their anxiety made them feel more comfortable in an unfamiliar situation. There is even a measure of comfort in an offered glass of water. Such comfort measures supported the clients' own abilities and assisted Mrs. Davidson in maintaining integrity and independence.

Trust also seems to contribute to the structure of caring. Trust may be defined as that relationship wherein the patient or client has confidence or faith in the nurse. He relies upon the nurse's integrity to accept him, his feelings and needs and to provide nursing care based on knowledge, skill and expertise. In order to be cared for, clients must have trust and confidence in the person helping them. Mrs. Davidson began to trust the nursing staff as she perceived their genuine concern for her situation. As the nurses interacted with her in a warm and open manner and their behavior reflected what she considered appropriate nursing responses, the level of trust she felt for the staff increased. Trust in itself is probably not a single function, as any number of factors in various mixes at different times may contribute to a trusting relationship.

In the situation just discussed, it would seem that certain qualities exhibited by the nurses facilitated a *trusting* client relationship. Some of the qualities perceived are *genuineness, acceptance* and *empathy*. Genuiness means that in response to the clients, the nurses accepted their feelings of frustration and anger in an open manner. The nurses' acceptance of the clients' feelings assisted in the development of a trusting relationship. Acceptance indicated the nurses had a warm regard for Mrs. Davidson as a person of worth, regardless of her feelings. Acceptance in the nurse-client relationship is defined as the nurse's acceptance of the client as a person and of all his feelings, negative or unpleasant, as well as positive. Empathy is the desire and attempt to understand another person and his perception of the experience. It implies sensing the meaning and feeling in another's communications, even if they are not explicitly stated. The nursing staff demonstrated empathy for Mrs. Davidson and her husband when they comprehended their anger and frustration and were able to understand and appreciate their emotions and actions. Achieving the qualities of genuiness, acceptance, and empathy is not possible in every instance of nurse-client relationships, not even possible completely in any one relationship, but they are components toward which nursing activities are directed. Their value is crucial because they contribute to the establishment of a trusting relationship, which, in turn, has been predicted as crucial for the continuity of caring.

Trust and comfort did not occur simply because the nurses meant well and wanted to help; their development was influenced by other factors as well. Mitchell[10] indicates that the past experiences and present situation of both nurses and clients as well as the current needs of the client have an important bearing on the development of a helping process. In addition, there are important tools and skills which a nurse brings to a relationship with a patient-client. These include knowledge, communication skills, technical expertise and oneself. They impact considerably upon the processes and activities of nursing and influence the contribution that trust and comfort make to professional caring.

The Structural Elements of Caring

The world of nursing phenomena is continuous, yet an attempt has been made to break it up into discrete parts and describe its functional unity, or how the structure of caring and its components are integrated and work together with a degree of internal consistency. Caring phenomena are composed of *structure* as well as processes and activities that nurses do for and with clients which contribute to the integrity and continuity of caring. Yet thus far, this author feels a sense of dissatisfaction with what has been theorized about caring. Certainly, a valid criticism of the structural-functional approach is that it is overly mechanical and can easily lead to tautologies. To break away from this circular path, British social anthropologists have used what they label as "structuralism". Levi-Strauss[12] maintained that the first step in scientific procedures is the structural study of a subject matter—be it social facts, linguistic facts, or other phenomena. He suggested that the construction of *binary* models would tell us more than the mere description of facts. His objective was to construct a model abstract enough for purposes of comparison, which would not only describe the given set of social entities, but also at the same time offer both contrast and illumination. Levi-Strauss built upon the elementary oppositions set in motion by the functions within his structures to derive the more complex, underlying "mentalist" structures with which he had dealt. However, the structure of a given phenomenon should be sought as closely as possible at the empirical level, at least for its present utility in the development of nursing theory. But the process of contrasting and explaining social entities is helpful in the interpretation and description of caring phenomena. For example:

> Mr. Kelly was hospitalized with pneumonia and had developed delirium tremens. He had been having hallucinations all day, shouting at the ceiling and warning away anyone who came near him. To protect him and others, he had been secured to his bed with a waist restraint. During the evening, he had to be moved into another room, and two nurses went to move his bed. "Get away, get away; save yourself, missy," he shouted. He became more and more agitated as the nurses wheeled his bed down the hall. He was shaking more violently than ever, and one nurse thought, "Why, he's frightened to death." She told the other nurse to stop; she put her arm around Mr. Kelly and began to talk to him in a quiet voice, soothing him as she would a frightened child. After a few minutes he became quiet and agreed to proceed to the new room. The nurse continued to sit by him for a while, telling him she would not let anyone harm him. He soon fell asleep.[11]

Mitchell indicates that the words the nurse used were not important. By becoming involved with the patient and by participating in his experience, her nursing care contributed to caring and the structure of caring as a structural entity. But suppose that instead of responding to the meaning of fear for the client, the nurse responded by becoming anxious that Mr. Kelly would injure himself or perhaps even harm her. If this has been the case, her response would have been quite different. Perhaps she would have called for assistance from an orderly and applied wrist restraints also. She might have administered a PRN sedative. Both of these actions would have implemented the original goal of the nurse—quieting Mr. Kelly down so he could be moved safely to another room. These processes or activities, had the nurse carried them through, would certainly not have made the contribution to the caring entity as clearly as her other previously described actions. Caring, even though a central and important part of nursing, does not always occur. Its opposite, *estrangement* from the patient, can also occur. When a nurse is estranged from her client, she cannot care because she is unable to relate to or to care for him. The opposite of being estranged is to find a person believable; this allows for caring to occur.

In analyzing the example that led to estrangement of nurse and client, we conclude with some hesitation that the safety of the patient and of the nurse are laudable and worthwhile goals of nursing care. If based on her professional knowledge and expertise the nurse made a decision and acted to ensure the safety of the client and herself in the process, few nurses would question her professional judgement. Yet, as previously indicated, this example of nurse-client interaction does not contribute to caring as it has been defined in this paper. The caring model that has been developed is *not* a stable, fixed system; its stability is only a hypothesis, not an established fact. By examining the contradiction of caring—estrangement—it can be seen that estrangement makes no contribution to the continuity of caring, which has been postulated should exist in nursing. Estrangement contradicts caring. Dealing with opposition and contrariety is useful in attempting to define the parameters of caring structure, although the use of oppositions in this instance falls short of a dialectical view. The opposed entities of caring and estrangement do not generate each other or necessarily clash, nor do they pass into each other in the process of being transformed into something else. At this point they just exist as empirical entities within a whole. This analysis has not answered the question of, "Why do nurses specifically care, or why do they estrange themselves from clients?" Yet these are intriguing questions. Not only should theories be phrased in ways that allow for prediction but the reasons why predictions occur should also be apparent.

If the contributions to caring which have been identified as trust and comfort are not an integral part of the nurse-client relationship, then it could be postulated, for example, that both caring and estrangement are generated from the social activities that occur in the nurse-client relationship. If in the preceding example, the nurse had been unable to establish a genuine relationship with the patient because she was not aware of her own negative and condemning attitudes toward alcoholics, she would not have been able to establish acceptance of him as a person. Without genuineness and acceptance, empathy—which is the desire and attempt to understand another person and his perception of experience—could not be established. This would contribute to the structure of estrangement—the condition of finding a person not believable.

Summary and Conclusions

Obviously, there are a number of limitations in this theory of nursing. The entire scope of caring needs systematic investigation with emphasis upon caring needs of clients and caring behaviors of nurses. Other methodologies need to be utilized that allow for a more dynamic analysis. Application must therefore be made to the observation of what nurses actually do and how critical decisions are made in nursing care to give a dynamic consideration of structural change in caring.

The value of this theory of nursing to the author is a *personal* one. The discipline required in the exercise of writing this theory of nursing has been considerable and has reaffirmed a belief that the study of caring phenomena is a serious and necessary challenge for nurse-theorists. Nurses obviously have a great deal to learn about caring and its effect upon clients. This theory of nursing, with its focus upon the entity of caring, is a beginning step toward exploration of the total dimensions of caring phenomena.

References

1. Evans-Pritchard EE: Social Anthropology: Past and Present. In Bohannan P, Glazer M: Highpoints in Anthropology. New York, Alfred A Knopf Co, 1973.
2. Jacox A: Research in Nursing—A Contemporary View. The American Nurse, September 15, 1976.
3. Harris M: The Rise of Anthropological Theory. New York, Thomas Y Crowell Co, 1968.
4. Radcliffe-Brown, AR: On the Concept of Function in Social Science. In Bohannan P, Glazer M: Highpoints in Anthropology. New York, Alfred A Knopf Co, 1973.
5. Ellis R: Characteristics of Significant Theories. Nursing Research, Vol 17, 3:217-227, 1978.
6. Andreoli K, Thompson, CE: The Nature of Science in Nursing. Image, Vol 9, 2:32-37, 1977.
7. Walker LO: Toward a Clearer Understanding of the Concept of Nursing Theory. Nursing Research, Vol 20, 5:428-435, 1971.
8. Kuhn TS: The Structure of Scientific Revolutions, 2nd ed. Chicago, The University of Chicago Press, 1970.
9. Leininger M: The Phenomenon of Caring—Caring the Essence and Central Focus of Nursing. American Nurses Foundation, March 1977, 2, 14.
10. Mitchell PH: Concepts Basic to Nursing, 2nd ed. New York, McGraw-Hill Book Co, 1977.
11. Myeroff M. On Caring. New York, Harper & Row, 1971.
12. Levi-Strauss C: Social Structure. In Bohannan P, Glazer M: Highpoints in Anthropology. New York, Alfred A. Knopf Co, 1973.

Caring: A Life Force

5

Em Olivia Bevis, R.N., M.A., F.A.A.N.

Caring is one of life's essential ingredients; it may be its most essential ingredient. Caring helps to insure that life goes on by producing primary groups and a positive environment for children and adults. Caring helps to prevent disease, promote health, heal or help the vulnerable, educate the population, and raise human relationships to satisfying experiences of pleasure, security, trust, growth, and positive activity. Love, hate, fear, happiness, anger, pleasure, or any other human emotion may have the growth-producing, energy-generating, motivating, and consistently positive effects of caring. All other human feelings have potentially negative effects as well as positive ones, but caring by its nature and definition is only and always positive.

Caring: An Art

Caring is a process and an art form. Just as Fromm[1] declares love is an art, so is caring. An art is a discipline with theoretical, philosophical, and practical aspects. To care skillfully without studying the philosophy and theory of care is to rely solely on one's instincts. We can do it, but on a trial-and-error basis. Something as important to life, as central to life's fulfillment as caring deserves thought, study, and practice. No pianist would think of giving a concert without studying and practicing the music. To pick out the pieces by ear and play them hit-or-miss would spell failure for most artists. Even pianists like Errol Garner who played by ear, practiced, thought about, and talked about the music. Playing does not just happen—it is a planned, worked at, thought about, practiced event. It is the rare person who can really care about others, about self, about things or events without the lifelong study of and commitment to caring.

An artist has several characteristics which distinguish him as an artist. First, an artist has dedication and commitment to the art. Second, an artist has knowledge of the theory. Third, an artist practices in a wide variety of expressions of art. Caring as an art requires all three of these elements: *commitment to caring* as an important aspect of life, lifelong *study of the theory and philosophy of caring* and continual *practice of caring* for and about people, events, and the progress of society.

True caring is infectious. It permeates all aspects of our life. Caring affects the choices we make about the use of time, what we do in our leisure time, the effort we put into our work, the priorities we set, and the relationships we choose or choose not to cultivate. Caring affects how we view ourselves or our own strengths, attributes, and characteristics. It affects our ability to give love and compliments, and to accept them. It molds and directs our hopes, dreams, visions, and influences our arrangement of life so that these futures come to pass.

Definitions of Care

Care and *cure* are derived from the word *cura,* which has a double meaning. Caring is used as *anxious exertion* as well as *carefulness and devotedness.* Both of these meanings influence the modern English use of the words care and cure, and are reflected in the definitions examined here.[2]

May offers the best definition of caring: "It is a feeling denoting a relationship of concern, when the other's existence matters to you; a relationship of dedication, taking the ultimate terms, to suffer for, the other."[3] Notice that he mentions suffering, and he names *dedication, mattering* and *concern* as essential elements. May seems right. *Caring* begins as a feeling, but because it is the feeling of caring it cannot remain only in the feeling domain. Caring compels the acting out of one's feelings. When something matters, we are willing to expend energy in structuring life so that positive things happen to and for the ones we care about. Caring demands that feelings be converted into behaviors and that the behaviors and feelings be accompanied by thoughts. The feeling of caring is not thoughtless; it is thoughtful.

Heidegger speaks of care as "the source of the will".[4] For him, the will is the driving force of life, and care is its source. He speaks of care as the basic phenomenon of human existence inclusive of the sense of selfhood. In other words, by not caring we lose our selfhood, our being, our will. In not caring our being disintegrates. Heidegger believes that conscience manifests itself as care. Therefore, while May sees caring as mattering, dedication, and being willing to delight in and suffer for, Heidegger sees it as equivalent to the will or the motivating force of life. They both seem correct and their definitions inclusive and not exclusive each of the other. I accept and use their definitions and elaborate on them in order to provide a clearer framework for my definition of caring which follows: ***Caring*** *is a feeling of dedication to another* to the extent that it motivates and energizes action to influence life constructively and positively by increasing intimacy and mutual self-actualization.

I propose that caring has four stages, namely: attachment, assiduity, intimacy, and confirmation. Each stage is attained by successfully completing tasks necessary to each stage. Caring becomes warped, nonfunctional, or stagnant when one or more of the tasks are not successfully accomplished; the mere nonaccomplishment of a task may stagnate the process, but the adulteration of a task changes the process to such a degree that it becomes something else, and is no longer caring.

The Purpose of Caring

Caring can be viewed by examining the purposes behind the behaviors of caring. Since all behavior is purposeful, it is well to examine purpose or motive. The purpose of caring is first, to facilitate mutual self-actualization. All other goals are subordinate to that overall purpose. Attaining one's full potential is life's most important goal. Most of us merely scratch the surface of what we are capable of achieving. Achievements in this sense may not only mean the producing of great books, or being president of the company, or chief of staff, or being tapped by Phi Beta Kappa. Achievement means developing capabilities—capabilities to know and to fully experience another human being, capabilities for patience, kindness, compassion, love, and trust, and capabilities to exercise one's latent psychic abilities, insights, imagination, and creativity. Finally, achievement is the capability to fulfill one's own ambitions, desires, goals, and dreams, so that one feels a satisfaction with one's life and the progression of it with the dedication and commitment which demands that something positive be done toward the direction of reaching full human potential.

There are other purposes underlying the behaviors of caring. As mentioned earlier, they are subordinate to the overall purpose of *mutual self-actualization.* They are:

1) To facilitate an improvement in the cared one's state, condition, experiences, and being.
2) To further the caring relationship.
3) To express feelings about the relationship.

Since purposes and motives are seldom single, some behaviors (by accident or design) fulfill two or all three purposes. Things that occur in our purpose area may affect the achievement of other purposes.

Factors Affecting Caring Behaviors

Caring is a universal phenomenon, a feeling that by its very nature evokes certain thoughts and compels certain behaviors in all cultures of the world. Probably, all people experience similar feeling states when they care. However, the way one thinks about caring and the way one who cares behaves are culturally conditioned and are affected by many variables. The experience of the feelings of caring (when raised to the level of thoughts and behaviors) go through a process of interpretation through language and acts that are symbols and manifestations of feelings that can only be expressed in ways that have been socially programmed. The consequences of these caring feelings, though many people probably have similar feelings, and the ways these feelings are described and/or acted out are through behaviors with cultural overlays that obscure and most often defy accurate comparisons. For this reason we will focus upon an "average" American framework. Whether an individual fits the description of caring thoughts, feelings and behaviors described here depends upon many factors. Deviations from the descriptions are normal expressions of individual variations affected by many variables, some of which are discussed here.

Culture

While caring is considered to be a universal human phenomenon, its expressions and activities are culturally conditioned and rewarded.[5] Social approval and social expectations depend entirely upon the unique cultural milieu in which the caring takes place. Whether a caring act is expected and approved depends upon the interpretation of that act through the screen of cultural overlay.

Therefore, while the basic influencing factor of caring is cultural conditioning, other factors also influence caring behaviors. Culture is an influence, in that it dictates how important caring is to the individual. Culture also influences how each factor is expressed and acted on and indeed, which factors will come into play. In the final analysis, culture controls how an act or behavior, once completed will be perceived and interpreted by the caring persons and by society at large. The following example of caring acts by mothers of three imaginary children demonstrates cultural influence on caring behaviors.

> Three little boys, one from Northern Europe, one from Israel, and one from America, were playing. They all fell and scraped their knees. They jumped up and ran to their mothers crying, while small amounts of blood oozed from the wounds and ran down their legs. The Northern European mother said, as she hugged her son, kissed him on the forehead, and wiped away his tears, "Don't cry now, be a little man; you are not hurt badly," (she emphasized sexual role programming, focused on the present, and on not showing emotions over pain). The American mother said, as she picked up her son, placed him in her lap and held him close while kissing him, "Don't cry now, it will be okay in a little while and heal before you know it. Let's put some antiseptic and a bandage on it," (she stressed the injunction not to cry, programmed optimism and a belief in science and medicine). The Israeli mother said, "Oh my poor baby," picked him up, kissed him multiple times, saying, "If only I had been watching you more carefully it wouldn't have happened...I wonder if all that bleeding means there is something wrong with your blood clotting?" (she stressed that someone was to blame and there must be some ominous meaning to the injury).

Each of these mothers cares for her son. Each expresses caring in ways approved by the culture, and in so doing transmits what is right and proper for caring. Social approval and expectations, or social conditioning is a primary factor influencing caring acts.

Values

Values are also culturally dictated. Values vary markedly from one individual to another within the same culture. Our value system is basic to our whole decision-making schema. Values dictate what we like, how important it is by order of priority, the choices we make about how to spend time, money, and energy. Motives, purposes, and goals are all influenced by our values. What we are willing to risk or give up in order to attain a goal is influenced by our values. Value is price. It is getting our money's worth, our energies' worth, or our caring's worth. "Is it worth it?" is the ultimate values question and is closely linked to caring.

Cost

A third factor that influences what we are willing to do in caring is the cost in time, energy, and money, as well as the cost in other relationships. In true caring we do not needlessly or unwisely expend time, energy, or money that will result in harm to self. In order to achieve a very important goal (for instance, saving a life), the caring person may hurt himself. However, in few circumstances is it necessary or desirable to hurt the self, for caring by definition is positive for both caring parties, and needlessly hurting or scarificing ourselves adulterates caring and turns it into a malignant force that is *not caring*. Martyrdom is not the material of true caring.

Exclusiveness

Another factor to be considered is exclusiveness. In true caring relationships, exclusiveness is something one passes through. If it remains as a permanent part of the relationship it is a negative factor and is therefore not caring. Other relationships are seen as necessary to the human condition, to growth, to stimulation, and to caring, and are therefore not sacrificed for a single exclusive relationship.

Maturational Level

The maturational level of individuals concerned in a caring relationship affects the quality and type of caring relationship entered into. Erickson[6] describes the stages of development as: 1) trust, 2) autonomy, 3) initiative, 4) industry, 5) identity, 6) intimacy, 7) generativity, and 8) integrity. In each of these stages the individual is capable of dimensions of caring relationships that were not available to him prior to accomplishing the tasks of that stage. The infant may not be capable of true caring relationships (whether or not this is so is a matter of conjecture because of the infant's lack of communication skills). The infant is generally a recipient of a parent who cares. With the development of autonomy and trust the basis is laid for true caring relationships. Caring relationships require that the unity of caring be outfitted with the integrity of individuality. In that way, autonomy is developed. If we skip either trust or autonomy we cannot truly develop caring relationships. Adolescents very often develop caring relationships to a point, and then adulterate them by surrendering their identity to each other so that the relationship becomes dependent. Mature people develop caring relationships more easily than others, for they have accomplished the developmental tasks that make caring possible.

Scripts

All children find as they begin to grow and develop that there may be conflict between their potential and their freedom to develop. Many children find it necessary to make decisions to fit the environment in which they live in order to survive. These decisions may be made before the child is equipped or prepared to make such important life resolves, yet they set the course for the child's future. The child receives these rules from parental figures, who in turn base the injunctions, rules, or scripts on their own fears, wishes, fantasies, self-esteem, and life decisions. Goulding[7] has listed ten major injunctions upon which individuals seem to base their decisions. From these ten injunctions, there are six that would directly affect the caring experiences of an individual. Our life decisions have tremendous impact and influence on our caring relationships. Identification and increased awareness of these decisions will allow an individual to examine them and to make re-decisions about his life and then, relationships with others. Life decisions create life patterns and are an important variable that will influence movement through the caring process. It may require time, energy, and possibly therapy to manipulate and change these variables.

Stress Levels

Stress levels affect people and the manner in which they care. For some, stress causes withdrawal and isolation, and therefore decreases the willingness of the person to allow caring feelings and behaviors to emerge. For some, stress promotes reaching out and establishing warm human contact so that caring behaviors are encouraged. People are generally ready recipients of caring from others during stressful times. Often, in such public places as buses, street cars, subways, airplanes, and airports, caring people converse with strangers who are under stress and who reveal intimate details of their lives. Under ordinary circumstances people would have to be in a much more advanced stage of intimacy before such self-revelation would occur. People who are sick and in hospitals are often open to caring relationships with fellow patients and health care providers that would be less likely to occur (at least as rapidly) were the stress factors less. People experiencing grief are usually open to caring acts from others. They allow more hugging, holding, kissing, acts of thoughtfulness and kindness, protection, and support than usual and from a wider variety of people, including people with whom they are in stages of caring that do not have such acts as central and usual behaviors. In stress, caring becomes a sliding continuum that moves freely into and out of behaviors that ordinarily move in an orderly procession through carefully perceived sequences.

Time

Time becomes an important influencing factor in caring only when it is in short supply. People facing leavetaking through moving away, war, or death tend to slip through the caring process at a more rapid rate. It is as if the fact of temporality, of finiteness, brings a realization of the value of the caring relationship and provides it with a vitality that brings to the fore the relative nature of time, so that movement through the process of caring occurs rapidly. It seems that people are willing to take more interpersonal risks, to trust more, to reveal more of themselves, and to believe in the veracity of the relationship more intensely when time is short. Under the constraints of time, people seek to take relationships as far as possible before time runs out.

Conversely, sometimes temporality provides the excuse for relinquishing the possibility of a caring relationship. The anticipation of pain in separation can make reluctant participants in caring because of the inevitability of the separation. Nurses, therapists, teachers, etc, are engaged in work that has vitality only if caring is present. But by the nature of their work, the relationship is from the very beginning, timebound. Unrestrained and uninformed capitulation into the caring process can lead to rapid burn-out.

Caring and Other Feelings and Processes

Many concepts are close to caring in nature and often are confused with it. These are *love, sex, intimacy, concern,* and *duty*. In order to truly understand caring thoughts, feelings, and behaviors, it pays to study these other similar concepts so that the whole construct has more meaning. The problem is that each of these concepts has characteristics in them which are part of others so that it is hard to delineate them. A brief discussion of these five feelings follows below.

Love

Love is probably the most global concept, and covers aspects of all the others. Separating love from caring is difficult, for love and caring are often seen as the same. Loving is a feeling. However, it can be expressed in caring and in noncaring ways. It can sometimes find perverse expressions. Some would argue then that unless it is positive, it is not true loving. Perhaps that is correct. However, love can be extremely selfish in its expression; caring cannot be. In the final analysis, love may defy theories; it may be too complex for definition. Though it is hard to separate the feelings from their expression, it may yet be done. Perhaps the careful explication of the nature of caring will separate caring from love so that the pure state of love may be more easily examined. This is not to imply that caring can be entirely separated from love. It cannot, for love is a large portion of caring.

Love is complex for English-speaking people because the word is used to express such a wide range of feelings. The Greek language has at least four words for love:

1) *Epithemia:* desire; implying lust and impurity; libido.
2) *Eros:* love of truth, beauty and goodness. It aspires to fulfill life and the spirit's yearnings.
3) *Filia:* brotherly love, affection, comradeship, friendship, neighborliness.
4) *Agape:* sacrificial love, altruism, unselfish, unconditional.

Essentially, *epithemia* and *agape* are incompatible. *Epithemia* implies impurity, selfishness, the supremacy of need even if the consequences may not lift one to higher planes; whereas *agape* is always unselfish, pure, and unconditional. *Eros,* too, is conditional, worth being measured by quality or beauty. *Eros* is an egocentric love, and contains the assertion of self-values, even if the values are noble, sublime visions and yearnings toward truth and beauty. For Americans, the concept of love is confusing because it incorporates the meanings of the four different Greek words, and as shown, these meanings are sometimes in conflict with each other.

Love is further compromised by its use as a sales gimmick. By the use of the word love, it can sell deodorants, mouthwash, toothpaste, and complexion soaps. On a deeper level, love sells home and family in ten-minute commercials sponsored by various religious groups. Love can influence duty and commitment as conditioned by parental injunctions. The giving and taking of love is equated with liking, friendship, sex, and jealousy. It is generally a nebulous, ill-defined, amorphous entity that is colored by hopes, dreams, aspirations, and guilt.

The important points to remember about the differences between love and caring is that with love, one may be altruistic and self-sacrificing by giving up one's own needs in the service of and to the benefit of another. In caring, both persons must be served. Even though we may delay gratification, unlike true love we do not permanently give up our own needs. The caring person does not abase himself. Attempts to unite with another at the expense of self or the other must by necessity be noncaring. However, this begs the question of the other forms love takes (*eros,* and *epithemia*) and how they can (by their goals and their nature) be in conflict with *filia* and *agape.* Caring is akin to *filia,* yet it has the unconditional aspects of *agape* without the self-sacrifice. Caring in emergencies can be altruistic and sacrificial, but in its everyday interaction it is not, for it is egalitarian.

Sex

Sex is one way people seek to overcome the sense of isolation and separateness. It can be a successful way if it is entered into through love. Sex, though, is a basic drive and as such is like Freud's itch that must be scratched. This is true insofar as humans are part of the animal kingdom and use sexual coupling to reproduce the species. But in humans, itching and scratching vastly oversimplifies the matter. As far as we know, humans are the only animals that have intercourse for the sole reason of pleasure.

Sex is a matter of pleasure and creative expression—an expression of caring, love, need, dependency, pity, desire, happiness, the desire for unity, or an escape from the prison of aloneness. It is covered by a multitude of mores, folkways, taboos, injunctions, instructions, theories, myths, and fantasies. Sex is used to prove one's masculinity or femininity, to prove one's sincerity, one's commitment, to shore up one's ego, to act out hostility. Sex is a means of communicating, or rebelling, or of caring. Sex can be one of the highest and most beautiful expressions available to human beings, or one of the lowest and basest.

Sex and caring are intertwined because sexual expressions of caring and tender feelings are inevitable in relationships between caring parties. As mentioned earlier, caring feelings *must* be acted upon, and sexual expression is simply one way caring feelings are expressed. How they are expressed is dependent upon the values, the expectations, the cultural mores, and folkways of the person's group, and on his parental injunctions.

One problem with labeling behaviors *sexual* is that it erroneously connotes an ultimate goal of copulation. Some sexual behaviors are expressions of sublime tenderness made physical, and have no other purpose than to give vent to caring feelings in ways that bridge isolation. The earliest and most familiar behaviors are those that are expressed in physical, non-genital ways and are felt by both sender and receiver as being sexual. For instance, the first tender acts humans receive are usually sexual: feeding at mothers' breasts, being stroked and petted all over, held and hugged close. These caring gestures, acceptable as *nonsexual* for children, are the same ones that are *sexual* for adults.

Sexuality, then, is a part of caring, and yet is a separate concept. There are many forms of sexuality without caring that are often confused with caring. Making love, or merely kissing, touching, holding hands, and hugging, are all ways of expressing love, caring, and tenderness. They are legitimate, healthy, noble ways, regardless of the gender of the caring parties, if they are expressions of true caring.

Concern

Concern is the concept that comes closest to being synonymous with caring. Concern is definitely a component of caring but only tells part of the story. It lacks the comprehensiveness of caring. Concern is not a process, though there are degrees of concern. Tillich used the term *ultimate concern* to describe faith.[8] His ultimate concern is very close to caring in that it is a feeling that one must act upon. It is caring about something, so that one must do something to improve the situation. Concern, however, is more closely aligned with worry, with being bothered about something. It also has an element of compassion, feeling with and for another's plight. Concern can be personal or impersonal, whereas caring is always personal.

Intimacy

Intimacy is a stage of the caring process and as such will be discussed only briefly. However, it is an independent concept and is often confused with caring. Intimacy as used here is two people sharing their innermost thoughts and feelings, and being comfortable in each other's presence.[9] It is not a euphemism for sexual intercourse. Rather, it is being welcomed in each other's inner room, the secret place people have within, where they store those hopes, dreams, disappointments, woes, fears, and shame that they do not want the general public or even fairly close friends to know about. In this respect, intimacy is the third stage of caring.

Intimate behaviors can be contextual. For instance, there is sexual intimacy, the intimacy of common goals, self-revelation intimacy, the intimacy of competition, the intimacy of hatred or enmity, the intimacy of fear, crisis, or oppression. These intimacies differ in duration, in purpose, in degree of accompanying commitment, in the presence or absence of caring and in the stage of caring. They also differ in strength, in frequency, and in the number of intimacies that we can manage at one time. It is not germane to caring to discuss each of these categories of intimacy.

Duty

Duty is a parental word full of shoulds and oughts, of guilt and responsibility. It certainly does not conjure up dancing and laughter, wine and song. It evokes vision of German soldiers belly-deep in the Russian snows, of nurses keeping vigil through long and arduous nights, of guard dogs patrolling deserted streets with policemen by their sides, and "him" marrying "her" because she is pregnant. Duty has been glorified in literature, extolled in poetry, praised by the clergy and raised to the status of a religion by the military. Duty are those acts *required* by feelings of responsibility. Duty may arise from caring feelings or may arise from injunctions that are family or culturally governed.

The Interpersonal Process

This is similar to the caring process in some respects, but vastly different in others. The interpersonal process is essentially a communication process that moves from approach through intimacy probably in much the same way as caring. There are, however, some essential components of caring that the interpersonal process does not have. First and most important is that caring has energy and vitality that demands that something be done to act upon those feelings, whereas the interpersonal process has no such drive or energy.

Second, the interpersonal process is the skill of communication. Communication skills are only one of several skills utilized in the caring process. Professional care providers may offer types of care such as pastoral skills, psychiatric therapy skills, nursing skills, and teaching skills as components of stage one and two of caring. Doing for others who cannot do for themselves, protecting the vulnerable, teaching the ignorant, keeping order and peace, giving energy to those who have insufficient amounts are all acts of caring in the first two stages. In the intimacy phase, this requires a person-to-person encounter on a more personal and more basic level than doing to and/or doing for, and at a much deeper commitment level than any uninvolved person could engender. The interpersonal process is a useful tool to enable the caring process to express itself.

Conclusion

This paper has presented caring as a life force, as motivation, energy, drive, will, and as a force *compelling action.* Caring is a feeling mandating relationship and because of the nature of the relationships, the feeling compels the caring person do certain things, complete tasks, and move through given stages. In that way, each person more fully reaches his potential—or to use Maslow's term, become self-actualized. In all races, religions, and in all historic times people have cared, have felt feelings of care, and have made covenants of caring. They have lived and acted out caring. In the expression of caring, its acts have differed, from time to time, from culture to culture, but most probably, the feelings have always been one of the great forces shaping the course of mankind.

References

1. Fromm E: The Art of Living. New York, Harper & Brothers Publishers, 1956, p 5.
2. Partridge E: Origins: A Short Etymological Dictionary of Modern English. New York, MacMillan Co, 1958, p 135.
3. May R: Love and Will. New York, Dell Publishing Co, Inc, 1969, p 300.
4. Heidegger M: Being and Time, translated by Macquanie J and Robinson R. New York, Harper & Row, 1962, p 242.
5. Leininger M: The Phenomenon of Caring. Part V, Caring: The Essence and Central Focus of Nursing. American Nurses' Foundation Nursing Research Report, February 1977, Vol 12, No 1, pp 2, 14.
6. Erickson E: Childhood and Society, 2nd ed. New York, Norton, 1963, pp 247-273.
7. Goulding R: New Directions in Transactional Analysis: Creating and Environment for Redecision and Change. In Progress in Group and Family Therapy. New York, Brunner/Mazel Publishers, 1972, p 107.
8. Tillich P: Dynamics of Faith. New York, Harper and Brothers Publishers, 1957, pp 1-30.
9. Davis M: Intimate Relations. New York, The Free Press, 1973, pp xviii-xix.

Some Issues Related to a Science of Caring for Nursing Practice*

6

Jean Watson, R.N., M.S.N., Ph.D.

Nursing: Humanistic and Scientific

Since the field of nursing is both humanistic and scientific, it is based upon what can perhaps best be described as a science of caring. Caring includes the actual processes and methods which effect positive health behavior changes in the patient/client. The caring process consists of those aspects of nursing that are intrinsic to the therapeutic interpersonal process between the nurse and the patient/client. The caring process in nursing encompasses an area of knowledge within the biophysical, behavioral, and social sciences and the humanities. A science of caring seeks to understand how health and illness problems relate to human behavior and how human behaviors influence health-illness outcomes. Nurses seek to understand and appreciate how people cope under conditions of both health and illness.

Some nursing leaders are currently developing a science base for the caring process. A science of caring must achieve a delicate balance between scientific knowledge and humanistic practice behaviors. The development of a science of caring is unique in that it encompasses both scientific results and the deeper values of quality of living and dying. Understanding the similarities and differences between science and the humanities will help to explain why both are important in nursing and why a science of caring is needed.

Science, generally neutral with respect to human values, has the capacity for methodological procedures, comprehensive generalizations, and accurate predictions. However, there are important functions which science cannot perform if for no other reason than it asks different kinds of questions from the humanities. Science as such is not concerned with human goals and values. Science is not necessarily concerned with individual experience and one cannot expect the sciences to keep alive a sense of common humanity.

The humanities, in turn, address themselves to a different problem, ie, to understand and evaluate human goals and experiences. The humanities are concerned with emotional responses to experiences

**This discussion is drawn from the author's book,* Nursing: The Philosophical Science of Caring. *Boston, Little, Brown and Co, 1979. (At the time of this Conference, this book was still on press.)*

and they look for individual differences and uniqueness. The humanities seek diversity and quality of human experiences. In the humanities, imagination and insight are validated from within the self. However, the humanities are also limited. They cannot give us predictable solutions to the problems of human nature. Humanities cannot provide us with the hard data that comprise the tested content for nursing.

Because of the similarities and differences between science and humanities, nursing often finds itself in conflict. In practice, nurses may tend to emphasize one and deny the other. But in spite of inherent differences there exists the possibility for a science of caring which approaches human problems from both perspectives.

A science of caring requires us to examine and strive to understand the meaning of actions and values that determine human choice in health and illness. The present and future task of the nursing profession is to identify, describe, and research the interaction of both perspectives. Further development of the foundation of the caring process can lead to expansion of a science of caring.

Carative Factors

The following factors are identified as a tentative foundation of the caring process in nursing that can lead to further development and research. These factors are labeled *carative factors* since they aim toward helping another person maintain or attain a high level of health or die a peaceful death. *Curative factors,* on the other hand, are directed toward curing a person of disease or pathology.

The ten carative factors which combine science and humanities to form a structure for studying the caring process are as follows:[1]

1) Formation of humanistic-altruistic value system.
2) Instillation of faith and hope.
3) Cultivation of sensitivity to self and others.
4) Development of helping-trust relationship.
5) Promotion and acceptance of positive and negative expression of feeling.
6) Utilization of scientific problem solving methods for decision-making.
7) Promotion of interpersonal teaching and learning.
8) Provision for supportive, protective and/or corrective mental, physical, sociocultural, and spiritual environment.
9) Assistance with human need gratification.
10) Allowance for existential-phenomenological forces.

Basic premises for a science of caring in nursing provide the foundation for the identified carative factors and a rationale for the utility of caring as a construct in nursing science. One of these basic premises is that caring (and nursing) has always existed wherever there was a society. There have always been some people in society who have been able to achieve a caring attitude and behavior. Nursing has historically and traditionally had a caring stance and responsibility to other human beings. Recent advanced education and research efforts have allowed nursing to combine its basic humanistic orientation with relevant science. Another premise is that there often has been a discrepancy between theory and practice, or between the scientific and humanistic aspects of nursing. A science of caring helps to combine and integrate the similarities and differences.

Some basic assumptions underlying the caring process are as follows:[1]

1) Caring can only be effectively demonstrated and practiced interpersonally.
2) Caring consists of basic processes between people which result in some sense of satisfaction often associated with human needs.
3) Effective caring results in health promotion and individual or family growth.
4) Caring attitudes allow for a person to be as he / she is now but also to actualize potentialities for becoming different in the future.
5) Caring is a "healthogenic" practice—more so than curing. One can cure a disease or illness, but the practice of caring integrates scientific with humanistic knowledge to promote health and provide ministrations to those who are ill.
6) A science of caring is therefore different from, but complementary to, a science of cure.
7) The practice of caring is central to the nursing profession.

Promotion and Acceptance of Positive and Negative Expression of Feelings

With the above brief introduction and overview to the essential carative factors, one specific carative factor will be developed; namely, the promotion and acceptance of positive and negative expression of feelings.[1]

This carative factor may not be necessary to identify separately for it is an inherent part of a helping-trust relationship. Since there is a justifiable theoretical and research base to validate the scientific merit of this factor for a science of caring, I chose to identify and discuss this as a separate carative factor, as a theoretical and research factor related to cognition and behavior.

Research studies[2,3] indicate that both a rational factor and a *quasirational* (affective) factor influence thinking, decision-making, and behavior. It is generally acknowledged that feelings and emotions play a central role in people's behavior. Knowledge of psychodynamics and group dynamics help to explain the power of the affective domain. The emotional or affective influence in behavior has been labeled as extra-cognitive,[4] nonrealistic,[5] and quasirational.[2] The emotional component has been theoretically acknowledged in social and behavioral science literature. Izard[6] maintained that emotions constitute the primary motivational system of human beings. Other theorists have emphasized the important role emotions play in organizing motivating the sustaining behaviors.[6] Mowrer claimed that, "emotions play a central role, in those changes in behavior, or performances which are said to represent 'learnings.'"[7]

Social psychologists have used theoretical notions of consistency,[8] balance,[9] and dissonance[10] to describe intrapersonal behavior. Explanations have usually involved a discussion about the balance between two thoughts that result in certain decisions and behaviors, or a balance attempt between thoughts and feelings.

It is a fairly acceptable notion that there is a level of intellectual understanding which is quite different from the emotional understanding of the same information. Rosenberg[8,11] articulated and researched the hypothesis that there may be a disjunction between what an individual knows and feels about the same topic. Affective-cognitive consistency is usually sought by an individual. An inconsistency between thoughts and feelings can lead to anxiety, stress, confusion, or even fear. It may alter understanding, influence attitudes, and contribute to behavior.

In an interpersonal situation, both cognition and affect are operating. Cognitions about a topic or health-illness event and the related feelings may explain whether individuals communicate smoothly, hear each other, listen to each other, and indeed establish rapport or trust with each other.

Focus on one's feelings and the non-rational emotional aspect of an event is most appropriate for nurses engaged in caring behaviors. The focus on thoughts and opinions regarding health-illness matters have been primarily dealt with in nursing situations. Focus on affective responses aroused during the process have often been neglected; however, feelings alter thoughts and behavior and need to be considered and allowed for in a caring relationship.

Each of us has a set of cognitions and feelings which affect our behavior. The cognitive component represents the intellectual content. The affective component represents our feelings about the content and is more difficult to grasp. The affective is often inferred from how one reacts toward a specific idea or event. It may also be directly expressed by the individual. For example: "I'm really angry," "I'm pleased," etc. The behavorial aspect consists of action tendencies. They are inferred from what a person says he or she will do or actually does.

Theorists have described communication as consisting of three components: cognitive, affective, and conative (behavioral). Social psychologists have used these same three components to conceptualize attitude. Various aspects of these components have been developed theoretically. Much research has been stimulated by these elements in attitude studies. In an attitude context these components refer to "certain regularities of an individual's feelings, thoughts, and predispositions to act toward some aspect of the environment."[12] All three elements are considered important in explaining social interaction. They operate in our perceptions of self, others, and our experiences.

Cognition and affect differ in the degree to which they alter behavior. The cognitive aspect of behavior may be easier to explain and understand than the affective. However, the affective component is considered a central component for understanding behavior and its meaning. Feelings are thought to have a powerful effect on behavior and thoughts. The result is sometimes considered to be irrational or impulsive. There may be no particular logical or cognitive explanation for certain responses. A person's thoughts and behavior may be guided by certain emotions not quite within one's awareness or realm of recognition.

It is theorized and supported with psychoanalytic principles that an awareness of one's feelings may eliminate some of the irrational aspects of feelings and actually allow one to have more control over thoughts and behavior. For example, we may get irritable or angry quite inappropriately without full awareness of the feeling and how it is influencing our behavior and thoughts. If we are made aware of the feeling we may understand what triggered the anger. We may accept the feeling as universal to others in similar situations. This may free us to respond to the feeling with a sense of relief and to respond to the situation in a more appropriate manner.

The separation of cognition and affect was reported by the ancient Greeks. It has been commonly referred to in popular terms as gut level feelings. This suggests that there are certain basic emotions having or needing no cognitive explanation. Certain irrational feelings and possibly irrational thoughts and actions may or may not be in a person's control, depending upon the level of awareness. A practice of caring must allow for, promote, and accept positive and negative expression of feelings in self and others. This focus improves the level of awareness and internal control over one's behavior and actions.

The affective component of an attitude has been reported to be that aspect which is emotionally satisfying to a person. This suggests that emotions are serving a need and the person seeks to maintain a balance between feelings, thoughts, and behavior. The psychological literature has established that a change in any one of the three components may cause a change in the remaining two components. In general, most theories have recognized both the affective and cognitive elements in explaining behavior. One theorist in particular, Rosenberg[8,10] has been concerned with the precise relation between the affective and cognitive components. Other theorists prior to Rosenberg concentrated on the rational, cognitive causes of attitude change. Indeed, cognition has been demonstrated to change affect.[10]

On the other hand, in relation to the carative factor which allows for and focuses on feelings, Rosenberg has been the only theorist to demonstrate that affect will change cognition. He has established that an attitude can be modified by changing the affective component, which in turn changes the cognitive component. Rosenberg's central hypothesis is: "The nature and strength of the feelings toward an object or person are correlated with the cognitions associated with the...same."[10] Rosenberg's research findings supported a consistency between the affective and cognitive components of an attitude.

Rosenberg's theory and findings have important implications for a science and practice of caring. There is little other empirical research support for the influence that emotions and feelings have over human lives, although feelings are considered an essential part of human make-up. This precludes the support from research on psychotherapy and behavior changes which are subject to many more complex variables and uncontrolled conditions than Rosenberg's work.

Nursing theories and practices are developed around human differences. Individual and group counseling and psychotherapy are based on feelings.[12] Therapeutic intervention, helping relationships, and trust development are oriented around focusing on a person's feelings. A major carative factor has been identified as acceptance and promotion of positive and negative expression of feelings as a core component of nursing.

Rosenberg's theory and research attest to the success of an emotional focus. His basic theory is that certain feelings can change the associated cognition. His research has demonstrated this effect. Additional studies support the importance of expressions of feelings.[8] In a clinical study by Yalom, successful group therapy patients were asked to recall some single critical incident in therapy which seemed to them to be a turning point. The most common type of incident reported involved the patients suddenly expressing strong negative feelings, ie, hatred or anger. The common characteristics of this critical incident were reported as follows:[8]

1) The person expressed strong negative affect.
2) The expression was a unique or novel experience for the person.
3) The feared and fantasized catastrophe associated with negative feelings did not occur.
4) Reality testing ensued in which the person realized that the affect expressed was inappropriate in intensity or direction or that the prior avoidance of affect expression was irrational; the person may or may not have gained some knowledge of the source.
5) The person was enabled to interact more freely and to explore more deeply.

In this same study the second most common type of critical incident also involved strong affect, but in these instances, positive affect. The incidents had the following common characteristics:[8]

1) The person expressed strong positive affect, which was unusual for him or her.
2) The feared, fantasized catastrophe did not occur; there was no rejection, deriding, or damage to others by the person's display of positive feelings.
3) The person discovered a previously unknown part of self, which resulted in a new dimension in relationships with others.

These findings, combined with the more rigorous controlled work of Rosenberg, assist us in validating the strong importance of allowing others to express negative and positive feelings without defensiveness, but rather with understanding and support for the expression.

The nurse should be supportive enough to permit such risk-taking in self as well as in others. In addition, reality testing can occur for both the nurse and the other person in relation to the appropriateness of the feelings for the situation or the inappropriateness of avoiding certain feelings. In turn, the helping relationship will be facilitated to a deeper, more honest and genuine level necessary in the practice of a science of caring.

If feelings can and do change thoughts and influence behavior, the science and practice of caring must be systematically attentive to people's feelings in maintenance and promotion of human health, and people's response to illness. Promotion and acceptance of feelings is a caring process that has some scientific validity, but also addresses people's emotional responses to experiences with which the humanities are concerned. As such, this carative factor allows for individual differences and uniqueness in understanding health and illness. At the same time, as nursing increases its knowledge base about human emotional needs and health-illness experience, a scientific knowledge base can develop that leads to predictable solutions to the problems of human nature. Such data can help to build a foundation for nursing as a science of caring.

References

1. Watson J: Nursing: The Philosophy and Sciences of Caring. Boston, Little, Brown and Co, 1979.
2. Hammond KR: Probablistic Functioning and the Clinical Methods. Psychological Review, 4:255-262, 1955.
3. Hammond K, Todd FJ, Wilkins M, Mitchell D: Cognitive Conflict Between Persons: Application of the 'Lens Model' Paradigms. Journal of Experimental Social Psychology, 2:343-360, 1966.
4. Scott WA: Rationality and Non-Rationality of International Attitudes. Journal of Conflict Resolution, 2:8-16, 1958.
5. Mack RW, Snyder RC: The Analysis of Social Conflict-Toward an Overview and Synthesis. Journal of Conflict Resolution.
6. Izard CE: Human Emotions. New York, Plenum Press, 1977.
7. Mowrer OH: Learning and Behavior. New York, John Wiley, 1960.
8. Rosenberg MJ: A Structural Theory of Attitude Dynamics. Public Opinion Quarterly, 24:319-340, 1960.
9. Heider R: Attitudes and Cognitive Organization. Journal of Psychology, 21:107-112, 1946.
10. Rosenberg MJ. An Analysis of Affective Cognitive Consistency. In Hovland, CI, and Rosenberg, MJ (eds): Attitude Organization and Change, New Haven, Yale University Press, 1960, pp 15-65.
11. Secord PF, Backman CW: Social Psychology. New York, McGraw-Hill Book Co, 1964.
12. Travelbee J: Interpersonal Aspects of Nursing. Philadelphia, FA Davis 1971.

The Meaning of Caring in the Context of Nursing

Kathryn G. Gardner, R.N., M.S.
Erlinda Wheeler, R.N., M.S.

7

Introduction

The concepts of support and caring appear distinguishable from each other, but are closely related. If caring is essential for an individual's growth and development, support may be described as a specific component of the caring process. Caring and concern are common terms used by nurses to describe support. However, to the nurse in the United States the term *support* may imply more specific nursing behaviors and interventions than the term *caring*. Nurses frequently write that they provide support to or for the patient, but they do not write that they provide caring.

In this paper, some observations about support and current perceptions about the meaning of support for nursing will be discussed. These ideas on the meaning of support have been extracted from a review of nursing literature, which provided a basis of our current research attempt to arrive at an operational definition of support in nursing. The method used in our pilot research study and some preliminary findings from the data analysis will be discussed. Perhaps this paper will stimulate further thought about the meaning of support, its relationship to caring, and methods that might be used to further study this concept.

Background

The investigators became interested in the meaning of support when we heard patients describe specific nurses as being *supportive.* Further observations showed that nurses in various practice specialities, such as medical, community health, and psychiatry, used the word *support* when they described nursing goals or interventions.

In reviewing some clinical data, the frequent use of the word *support* to describe nursing behaviors was surprising. In one observation from 35 psychiatric patients referred to community health nursing, 12 of them had "supported patient" written as a nursing order. In asking staff nurses what they meant when they stated that patients needed support, they were surprised and embarrassed when they could not give a simple, clear answer. The nurses' answers were long, usually involving a description of a particular patient's needs in detail, and did not suggest any generalized or consistent nursing behaviors. At the end of this description, the nurses would usually state that support was an important aspect of nursing care, but denoted certain nursing behaviors or expectations that could not be consistently stated.

A review of the nursing literature on support revealed that nurses regard support as an aspect of their nursing care.[1] The literature indicated several variables which might influence a nurse's ability to give support. Among these were the emotional and personal concerns of the nurse, the amount of time the nurse usually gives to patients, her knowledge, and skills (usually described as communication and interactional skills), and the receptiveness of the patient.

The frequent use of the term *support* in nursing practice and nursing literature and the obscurity of its meaning presented a dilemma. If support does not have a specific meaning to nurses, why is it used to describe interventions in nursing care plans and in writing nursing orders? The lack of a consistent and operational definition of support in nursing may be due to the fact that nurses have, by tradition, done and practiced a number of things by intuition, relying on experience as their guide. Only in the past few decades have nurses started to do research to expand their own body of knowledge. Therefore, many of the terms used in nursing practice have not been operationally defined or taught.

Concepts and Studies About Support

The term *support* is frequently used in the fields of psychiatry, psychology, and sociology, and some nurses may have adopted in part, if not totally, these usages and meanings. However, definitions of support in these fields are also diverse and often vague. In psychiatry and clinical psychology, the meaning of support or supportive therapy is more consistent than in other fields. It is used to define a specific kind of therapeutic relationship aimed at strengthening or reinforcing a patient's adaptation and ego functioning. Techniques commonly used in this type of therapy are increased activity, emphasis on the present and not the past, directiveness, a focus on problem-solving, and at times, advice giving.

To nurses, support seems to imply a subjective involvement. The opposite of support is associated with the technical aspect of nursing care or nursing skills. In the nursing literature, support has often been correlated with strengthening and adapting. The nurse, in supporting the patient, assists him in becoming stronger and adapting to his current life. These ideas of support correlate to a degree with the psychiatric definition of support or supportive therapy. Both definitions are concerned with the strengthening of the patient's ability to function; both are concerned with adaptation.

Certain nursing behaviors used to assist the patient to become stronger have been extrapolated from nursing literature: 1) the nurse demonstrated that she was available to the patient; 2) the nurse was able to communicate to the patient, verbally and/or nonverbally; 3) the nurse helped the patient to express his feelings; 4) the nurse engaged in problem solving with or for the patient; 5) the nurse assisted the patient in maintaining control; 6) the nurse helped the patient to make decisions; 7) the nurse conveyed understanding to the patient; and 8) the nurse gave information and/or explanations to the patient. Although each of these nurse behaviors was identified in the literature by several authors, all of them were not consistently listed by the majority of the authors.[1]

In a study by Pearlmutter,[2] salient emotional supportive behaviors identified were to regulate affect, receive or elicit expression of feelings, and provide control over the patient's behavior. Pearlmutter studied the meaning of emotional support by utilizing a questionnaire comprised of three selected patient situations, and asked 125 medical-surgical nursing staff to describe how they viewed the patient situation and what emotional support behaviors they would employ in the situations. Pearlmutter listed six categories of emotional support behaviors: assessing, intervening, communicating, conferring and coordinating, referring and securing resources, and recording.

Although identification of these nurse behaviors does not quickly lead to a clear definition of support, they are enlightening. Most of these behaviors assume that the nurse is able to interact and communicate with and to relate to the patient. From these behaviors it can be hypothesized that support means effective, goal-directed nurse-patient communication, which assists the patient in adapting to his current life stresses. The concept of strength is implicit in these nurse behaviors. A tentative working definition of ***support*** for nurses is extracted from those *behaviors aimed at helping the patient to maintain, restore, or increase his strength in order to enhance his ability to interact and adapt.* The nurse may strengthen the patient by assisting him to obtain or maintain control over himself, by helping the patient to recognize that he is a person of individual worth, and by helping the patient to utilize the resources available (this would include drawing upon the nurse's strength). From studying these behaviors it can also be surmised that nurses usually view support as being a psychological or emotional response—support which is centered around improving the patient's emotional state. Although physical care measures (especially comfort measures) are sometimes mentioned by nurse-authors under the rubric of support, physical care is more often viewed by nurse-authors as an adjunct of support. In the area of physical support, nurse behaviors are aimed at increasing a patient's comfort and control. However, in a study by Funkhouser,[3] it was concluded that nurses perceive the quality of the physical care as positively correlating with the quality of psychological support given.

In addition to physical and emotional support, there is some evidence in nursing literature that nurses also view support as being within a social context—that is, assisting the patient to remain or become socially integrated. However, compared with the emotional and physical aspects of support, social support has been given less significance. Two nurse-authors, Goldsborough[4] and Ujhely,[5] have written that one function of nursing care is to encourage social interactions and to serve as a socializing agent. Also, several nurse-authors have discussed another important nursing function, which is to work with families.

In contrast to the field of nursing as a whole, the nurse as a social therapist or agent is more accepted in the area of psychiatric nursing. Therefore, mutual withdrawal (the reciprocal decrease of interactions between the patient and nurse) has been long recognized as a problem in psychiatric nursing. Some nurse behaviors that encourage socialization are: 1) the nurse engages in social interaction and activities with the patient; 2) the nurse acts as a resource person; and 3) the nurse acts as a communication liaison between two parties on behalf of the patient. In the area of social support, the nursing activity is aimed at strengthening or maintaining the patients's social network.

The importance of support to health maintenance or promotion has recently been given attention. Caplan[6] believes that social support acts as a buffer against diseases and assists the person in maintaining health. Some research studies have suggested that lack of social support is disease-producing, and social support serves as a protective factor against disease etiology. This protective function of social support seems especially relevant in the presence of stressful situations.[7] Socially supportive environments are usually thought of as being health-promoting. The importance of social and emotional support is often viewed as a significant factor in determining the success of crisis resolution. Support seems to be one variable which may influence a person's susceptibility to, and rate of recovery from, various diseases. Within this theoretical framework, it becomes evident that nurses must further investigate the meaning and implications of support in their practice. Nurses are usually viewed as a critical component in the health treatment milieu and seem to be the most logical health professional to give support when it is needed and not supplied by the community or social system.

The concept of support should not be examined exclusively in the context of the nurse-patient relationship. It must also be studied in the interaction of the environment or milieu with the patient. Moos[8] included support as a subscale in his instrument which measures the social climate of psychiatric hospitals. This instrument, the Ward Atmosphere Scale, has been readapted to measure the social climate of jails and families. According, to Moos, his subscale support measures the concern for others in the milieu, the amount of helpfulness in aiding each other to resolve personal difficulties, and the amount of open communication. In a study by Turner,[9] it was found that patients felt more supported in a hospital milieu that had a functional nursing organization. Turner measured the amount of support that patients felt by interviewing them and by using an instrument which determined their ego identity. He described a supportive milieu as one that is "identity reinforcing". Turner's study (which to our knowledge has not been replicated) indicated that nurses are accurate when they state that their nursing influences the amount of support patients receive while in the hospital.

To aid in understanding and investigating the concept of support in nursing, an ego psychology theoretical framework may be helpful. In writing about human development, Erikson[10] hypothesized that an individual's ego progresses through the successful resolution of phase specific developmental sequences, and accidental crises. Thus, the growth of the individual's personality and his adaptation to society is particularly dependent on the reinforcement and help he has received when he is vulnerable and/or in a state of crisis. A crisis by definition implies a state of disequilibrium or vulnerability. At the time of disequilibrium or vulnerability, the interaction of the individual and his environment becomes critical. If the individual is aided to maintain or enrich ego functioning, then personal growth is likely to occur. Support can be conceptualized as those behaviors which are directed towards facilitating or maintaining the growth and integrity of the ego. The ego can be viewed as a unifying executive structure monitoring biological drives, cognitive processes, social demands, affective expressions and interpersonal interactions. According to nursing literature, the avenues most likely for nurses to use in giving support are problem solving behaviors and emotional acceptance, as well as physical care and social interactions.

Care and Support Relationships

The relationship of support to caring is a relatively unexplored territory. Care is often used to describe support. However, caring many be a prerequisite to support, and as such, it may not be an essential element of support *per se.* The differences between support and caring may be that support is more goal-directed than caring. Support may encompass behaviors employed by one person to strengthen the self-caring ability of the other person. Depending on the needs of the individual, support may be given over a short or long period of time. A person experiencing a crisis may require supportive measures over a short period of time, while a person with a long-term disability or disease—such as schizophrenia or cerebrovascular accident—may need prolonged support.

An unanswered question is: "Does one need to care in order to provide support?" It seems to be both theoretically and practically impossible to offer support without at least initially caring. Perhaps this question leads to more precise questions regarding the relationship of caring to support: "How much caring is needed to provide support?" and, "To what object is the caring directed?" In brief interactions it may be that minimal caring is needed to give support to another person. Initially, caring may not need to be directed to the object which requires support. For example, to initially give support, a nurse may need to care about herself and her work but not necessarily care for the patient as an individual. The motive for caring may be outside the nurse-patient relationship, particularly when the nurse first provides support. However, in a similar situation it would also be apparent that support for the patient could not be sustained unless the nurse also starts to direct her caring to the patient.

In a long term nurse-patient relationship, the caring process will need to develop in order for support to continue to occur. Caring in these relationships may become a reciprocal process, while support may remain unilateral. Support is provided or given to a person who is in need of it. Caring would seem to increase as more support is made available to the patient.

In our culture, support is a purchasable item. Individuals who have exhausted their usual familial and social resources are able to obtain support, and as a consequence, also obtain a limited amount of caring through paid services. Psychiatrists, clinical psychologists, social workers, ministers, and nurses are all professional persons paid to provide support. Individuals with a health problem who are in need of support from professionals are likely to receive it from nurses. Nurses are more accessible to them than other health professionals, and nurses have a long history of viewing themselves as providers of support.

The first project consisted of a two-part questionnaire. This questionnaire was sent to medical, surgical, and psychiatric staff nurses employed in a northeastern university hospital. The rationale for selecting these three groups of nurses was that all of the reported research on support had been done with either medical and surgical nurses or psychiatric nurses. One question we hoped to begin to answer was, "Did nurses in each practice specialty view the meaning of support differently?" If the answer to this question is affirmative, then supportive behaviors cannot be generalized from one specialty to another in nursing. The importance of social support to the practice of psychiatric nursing seems to indicate each specialty in nursing may view support differently.

The first part of the questionnaire asked nurses to describe an incident in which they gave supportive nursing. This critical incident technique was utilized because it is one method to document behaviors which may lead to an operational definition. The critical incident technique has been used successfully to determine other behaviors, such as combat leadership behaviors. By using this technique it was assumed that the nurse could write and report a critical incident by acting as her own observer. This assumption seems to be justified in that nurses have been taught to be observers of human behavior. The technique has proved successful in that it has begun to provide a rich source of data. The data were analyzed by one investigator listing all the behaviors described in the written incidents and placing each incident in one or more proposed categories of support: physical, social, or emotional. The other investigator blindly judged the first investigator's listing of supportive behaviors and categorization of incidents of physical, social, and emotional support. Agreement between the two raters was 98%.

If the lack of support is perceived by health providers as a health problem, then the provision of support should become a goal. The nurse, as a representative of the health professions, may be paid to provide support to patients whose usual support is undermined by illness or who are otherwise unable to obtain it in adequate amounts.

If these ideas about support and its relationship to caring are accepted as workable distinctions, then both support and caring become critical concepts for nursing to investigate. To date, little work has been done by nurses to scientifically investigate the concept of support. The work that has been done has been exploratory and descriptive. The few (we believe six) published studies reported in the past ten years by nurses have been neither replicated nor built upon.

In attempting to investigate this concept, the critical and perhaps most difficult task was to determine the most appropriate research design. With no clear and agreed-upon methodological approach available, a decision was made to try to build on two methods that have been used previously. The remainder of this paper will describe our design and share some of our preliminary findings.

Current Research of Investigators*

In order to build on the research ideas and findings of other authors, an extensive review of nursing literature was conducted. A list of all the words that have been used to describe support by nurses was made, with a total of 51 identified. Then a list of all nursing behaviors that were described as being supportive was made. These two lists became a part of the basic design for our first two pilot research projects.

In the second part of the questionnaire, all the words that had been previously used by nurses to describe support were listed in alphabetical order. The subjects were asked to rank each word on a four-point scale according to the level of its importance in supportive nursing, and to categorize each word according to the phase of the nursing process: assessment, planning, implementation, and evaluation, or general attitude. Several reasons for choosing this method were: 1) this design builds on two other reported research studies, one which asked respondents to give synonyms of support,[11] and another one which asked subjects to rank the importance of ten previously selected words to the concepts of support;[12] 2) in two reported studies, the authors discussed relationship of support to the nursing process but collected no data on this relationship; 3) by determining the mean and standard deviation of the ratings of each word and conducting a factor analysis, it was hoped that some theoretical and behavioral inferences could be made in regard to the definition of supportive nursing; and 4) it was anticipated that some beginning inferences could be drawn regarding whether nurses in different specialities viewed the meaning of support as being different or the same.

In collecting the data from this questionnaire, some interesting responses were received. Out of 382 questionnaires, 99 were returned—approximately 25%. Some nurses stated that they spent at least two hours completing the questionnaire. Although a few nurses became hostile because of the demands

**This study has been partially supported by funds from the University of Rochester, School of Nursing, Alumni Research Seed Fund.*

of the questionnaire, most were surprised that they could easily write a description of an incident when they gave support. The nurses, however, had more difficulty defining the meaning of support. The few hostile responses centered primarily around the idea that support was an inherent part of nursing practice and did not need to be defined. The low percentage of response may reflect the unexpected difficulty of the questionnaire. Although the length of time needed to respond may reflect the difficulty of the questionnaire, it may also reflect the importance that nurses give to support. The nurses who took the time to respond may be a biased sample in that they view support as being more important in their nursing practice than those who did not complete the questionnaire.

Another interesting aspect of the data collection was that some administrators, such as head nurses and clinical faculty, questioned the investigators as to how support was different from nursing care. Although staff nurses were verbal in their responses, only one asked this same question. This discrepancy may mean that support is viewed differently by those nurses who practice and those nurses who mainly teach and administer.

The preliminary analysis of our first study, using the critical incidents written by staff nurses practicing in medicine, psychiatry, and surgery, has been thought-provoking and stimulating. At this point, the data appears to have given us a few answers and has raised many questions pertaining to the staff nurses' perceptions of the meaning of support. For the purpose of sharing some of our first steps in understanding this concept, these data will be discussed.

Eighty-four staff nurses described 90 critical incidents in which they gave supportive nursing. Of these nurses, 35 were practicing in medicine, 25 in surgery, and 24 in psychiatry. Forty-three supportive behaviors were identified from the incidents. Nearly all of the incidents described some form of communication between the nurse and patient. Twenty-seven out of the 90 incidents, or 30%, mentioned communicating to the patient's families; 8 incidents, or 9%, mentioned communicating with other staff on behalf of the patient. The number of incidents mentioning communication with the family seems encouraging in that the respondents were simply asked to describe an incident in which they gave supportive nursing.

Each incident was categorized as physical, emotional, or social support. Physical support comprised those nurse behaviors centered around planning and implementing physical care; social support comprised behaviors aimed at increasing the patient's social integration and use of resources; and emotional support comprised behaviors aimed at improving problem solving ability and enhancing the patient's emotional state of wellbeing. Each incident can involve one to three categories. Ninety-three percent of the incidents were categorized as giving at least emotional support; 33% were categorized as giving at least social support; and 24% as giving at least physical support. Eleven incidents, or 12%, described all three categories of support. Seven incidents, or 8%, described physical and emotional support; and 18 incidents, or 20%, described social and emotional support. No incidents described both physical and social support. An example of an incident that mentioned physical, emotional, and social support follows:

> I had a young patient with terminal cancer. He was admitted several times over a six-month period. I feel that I established good rapport with the patient and his wife and both related to me more than the other staff. I feel this was accomplished by taking time to sit and wait for the patient to ventilate if he felt the need to. I also talked with his wife out of the room and found her needing to talk away from her husband. I provided support by listening to his wife discuss financial, emotional, and family problems. As the disease progressed, the patient required more physical care, and, as the family wished, we assisted them in giving most of the care. Discharge planning involved a public health nurse. He did not qualify for organized home care so I contacted many charities and organizations to borrow needed equipment for home use.

Still another example of an incident that focused on emotional support was:

> A patient was exhibiting neurological deficits, imbalance, and slurring of speech which brought him to seek medical attention. The day I was his nurse, I spent approximately 45 minutes with him discussing his symptoms, and his worries about the future. My role as a listener proved to be very supportive because the patient verbalized his feelings of frustration, fear, and inferiority. Verbalization of these feelings resulted in the patient feeling some relief. I then pointed out his many assets and talents that still remained with him (writing ability, education, intellect, experience in his area of work). He voiced his appreciation for my taking the time to listen to him and then discuss his feelings. I felt this intervention was supportive.

From a review of the incidence provided by the 84 respondents, seven behaviors were listed more than 20% of the time. Since each respondent may have illustrated a number of supportive behaviors, the following percentages do not total 100%.

TABLE I

THE EIGHT MOST FREQUENT BEHAVIORS IN THE CRITICAL INCIDENTS AS EXPRESSED BY A PERCENTAGE OF THE RESPONDENTS

Behavior	Percentage of Response
Helping patient to cope with feelings	39
Talking with/to patient	32
Sitting with patient	31
Giving information	27
Listening	26
Doing specific physical comfort activities	21
Touching patient	20
Coordination of care	20

These findings suggested some agreement with Pearlmutter's[2] work on emotional support. She found that the most important need that nurses perceived was the need for patients to express feelings, and an important intervention (behavior) was for the nurses to receive and elicit expression of feelings. Another important behavior from the Pearlmutter study was for the nurse to assist the patient in regulating affect and to promote a positive emotional climate.

A further examination of the frequency of the behaviors mentioned by the three nursing specialty areas also gave interesting data, as follows:

TABLE II

BY SPECIALTY NURSING GROUPS, THE EIGHT MOST FREQUENT BEHAVIORS IN THE CRITICAL INCIDENTS AS EXPRESSED BY A PERCENTAGE OF THE RESPONDENTS

	Percentage of Response in Each Group		
Behavior	Medicine	Surgery	Psychiatry
Helping patients to cope with feelings	34	32	54
Talking with/to patients	31	48	16
Sitting and spending time with patients	37	32	20
Giving information	34	44	0
Touching patients	14	32	17
Listening	26	36	17
Doing specific physical comfort activities	17	40	8
Coordination of care	20	28	12

Although the number of subjects in each group was too small to draw any definite conclusions, there seems to be a tendency for some supportive nursing behaviors to be perceived differently in each specialty group. Of particular interest is the response that psychiatric nursing does not view giving information as supportive. Another interesting finding is the importance that surgical nursing gives to physical care in describing support. If the meaning of support is interpreted differently by nurses in different practice areas, it is clear that this concept needs further study and scientific inquiry.

These findings are generally consistent with previous studies, ie, support is viewed by nurses to be primarily in the area of emotional support. Social and physical support, at this point, seem to be secondary to helping the patient cope with his emotional state or feelings. Although physical care measures are an important part of nursing practice, nurses, exclusive of surgical nurses, may not view these activities primarily as being supportive. At this time, there is little evidence that nurses view their practice as encompassing the area of social support. Perhaps nurses in a different setting, such as a nonacute or a rural setting, would view social support differently.

A limitation of the research design was that it required individuals to assess, judge, and describe behaviors as yet not investigated, which have a limited theoretical basis. An advantage of this design is that it is an efficient and relatively inexpensive way to obtain data that may lead to better theoretical premises and research designs to define the meaning of support. It is hoped that this research will lead to more effective descriptive designs, and eventually to some quasi-experimental and experimental designs on the meaning and effect of supportive nursing. The relationship of support to caring in nursing can only be investigated after these concepts can be operationally defined.

In our society, where computers will soon revolutionize health care delivery services, it seems imperative to study constructs such as caring and support. If not better understood, these concepts may be relegated to a less important place in the provision of health care. It is our opinion that these concepts must be understood, for their application represents the essence of nursing tradition and practice.

References

1. Gardner K: Supportive Nursing: A Critical Review of the Literature. Journal of Psychiatric Nursing and Mental Health Services, 17:6-10, 1979.
2. Pearlmutter D: Emotional Support Is—A Descriptive Survey. Journal of the New York State Nurses Association, 1:15-19, 1974.
3. Funkhouser GR: Quality of Care, Part I. Nursing, 12:22-31, 1976.
4. Goldsborough J: Involvement. American Journal of Nursing, 69:66-8, January, 1969.
5. Ujhely G: Determinates of the Nurse-Patient Relationship. Springer Pub Inc, 1968.
6. Caplan J: Support Systems and Community Mental Health. Behavior Publications, New York, 1974.
7. Murawski B, Penman O, Schmitt M: Social Support in Health and Illness: The Concept and its Measurement. Accepted for publication in Cancer Nursing.
8. Moos R: A Social Ecological Perspective on Medical Disorders. In Whittkower, Warnes E: Psychosomatic Medicine: Its Clinical Application. New York, Harper & Row, 1977.
9. Turner RJ: Social Structure and Crisis: A Study of Nursing Organization and Patient Adjustment. Community Mental Health Journal. 4(Winter):285-292, 1966.
10. Erikson EH: Childhood and Society. New York, Norton Publishing Co, 1950.
11. Stockwell M, Nishikawa H: The Third Hand: A Theory of Support. Journal of Psychiatric Nursing-Mental Health Services, 8:7-10, 1970.
12. DeYoung C, Dickey B: 'Support'—Its Meaning for Psychiatric Nurses. Journal of Psychiatric Nursing and Mental Health Services.

Part II — 1979

Analysis of Caring Behaviors and Processes

Second National Caring Conference

March 22, 23, 1979
University of Utah
Salt Lake City, Utah

Care, Culture, and Praxis

8

Michael J. Higgins, Ph.D.

Purpose

This paper is an attempt to find a common epistemological framework for nursing and anthropology. Why start at this level, and not at some pragmatic level of fieldwork and health care delivery? I believe that if we understand the pragmatic level, this understanding can become lost due to a lack of epistemological insights. I am not saying that beliefs determine behavior, but that those in nursing and anthropology do not understand the nature of our own behavior and need a new language to account for what we are doing as nurses and anthropologists. We have a tremendous amount of information about what different people's behavior indicates about their states of health and illness; however, when we wish to legitimize this information, we enter into a scientific discourse that neutralizes both our actions and the histories of groups of peoples we wish to learn from and materially aid. It is this double bind of the health practitioner I wish to address.

The Critical Overtones

We as health practitioners have some material wealth and useful power; however, we let that power be neutralized by accepting the ideological constraints of the dominant powers within our own social systems which dictate to us the terms of our means of action. If our hopes and programs in the area of multicultural health care systems are to be meaningful, we have to confront and redefine the domain of meanings in terms of our own history of labor. That is, we need to go outside the constraint of bourgeois ideology which attempts to grab the possible universal claims of science as their own products. Thus, until we know that we mean, the deck is stacked against us.

What are these constraints upon our actions? They primarily have to do with the opposition between our understanding of how people live and how people's actions get misused in the public or political domain. From the depth of our studies as health anthropologists, we know that health care systems work within the contexts of peoples' real lives and have only short-term effectiveness. However, the transmission of such ideas into general public discourse becomes a message about holistic health. Thus, the history of such peoples as the Navajos or the people of New Guinea and their successes in health care become a commodity in the chic department stores of health care for the middle income groups of our society. This derives from two related processes: the split reality of our own social system and our avoidance of that reality when we attempt to place our findings within the context of public discourse.

Let me attempt to explain what I mean by a split reality in our social system. It is what Sartre has called the opposition between existence and essence. A careful reading of the evolution of the structure and function of the human nervous system indicates that the ability to separate existence from essence has been part of our general human capabilities and is the common basis to the range of human symbols. However, the acting out of this human construct differs in the context in which humans find themselves and the ones they create for themselves. It is this type of human reality which becomes split within stratified state systems and most intensively split within an industrial capitalism.[1]

What then is the nature of this split reality within capitalism? The human division of the world into we/they and I/others becomes expressed as the difference between the individual and society within capitalism or for that matter, any stratified state system. This separation becomes the basis for the debate over the importance of the self in opposition to behavior, the group to society or society to culture. Sometimes these oppositions are referred to as the differences between the ideal and the real or the splitting of people's behavior into public versus private spheres of action. This way of thinking produces what Geertz referred to as the layering concept of human behavior: at one level we are biological, the next personal, then societal, and then cultural. Such assumptions also nicely match the division of the study of human behavior. Implied in all these splits is the assumption that the real—an empirically demonstrable phenomenon—is contained within the actions of particular persons; whereas the collective goal or ideal of a social system are to be found within the structures of that system. Thus we get a picture of people devoid of hopes while at the same time suggesting that somehow society or culture expresses somebody's hopes and ideals at some unstated time and place. If the real is the behavior of people and society, and if culture is the locus of hope or ideals of that real behavior, then what is the context of people's behavior? This may sound confusing. It is obvious that real people have real hopes and ideals and that society and culture are reflections of these patterns. I agree, except how we as health practitioners and health anthropologists have chosen to express that message results in the opposite means. Our descriptions of people tend to be statements about what people existentially face, while our concepts about that behavior tend to reflect what we ideally would like these people to be.

The Feminist Dilemma

Let me try to explain this by using a concept of private and public behavior that has been developed by feminist scholars. These scholars have stressed that historically it seems a pattern has developed in which women have been placed within the private sphere, which has been separate from the political and economic public world of males. As long as women were kept out of the public world, they were also kept away from any meaningful sources of power. Though I am aware of the realities of powerlessness among women, this conceptual split has always bothered me. It implies that the private world is a real world filled only with the drudgery of mundane labor and maintenance action; whereas the public world is the arena in which the ideals and goals that one seeks are to be found. I feel that, in fact, it is the opposite—it is the private sphere of action where the hopes and goals are constructed and the public sphere is where the "real" is confronted. It is the private sphere where the "hope fors" are constructed and the public sphere where they become hoped against. What all these conceptualizations do regardless of their orientation is to leave intact the historical contexts necessitating confronting such realities—the process of individual and collective alienation that maintains and reproduces the capitalist social system. So long as participants in the system do not know the public from the private in their own social system, they are hardly threatening to that system. Equally important is that if we cannot tell about our own social system, how are we ever going to understand other social systems? Crucial to an understanding of care is to know what happens to a process of caring within a social system based upon the alienation of people's creative actions, which include those of caring. Primarily, alienation is the process of separation of people from creative control over what they produce. Thus, if we wish to avoid this process in the training of people who can care, we need conceptual tools that can allow us to confront the reality of the process of alienation.

How then, do we address the process of alienation within our own social system? Make no mistake about alienation, for this is the labyrinth from which emerge the glaring social pathologies of our modern times. If we look outside the limited logic of cultural relativism, we see that the social systems from which we seek to learn something cannot provide us with such insights because we have placed them within the overall context of our industrial system. First, we destroy people; then we ask them to share their spiritual world with us so we can avoid the guilt of our own history. Until we face that history, we will remain the guardian of a liberal morality that has little meaning in the current context of the world in which we live. How do we face our own history? We need to construct a new scientific discourse that addresses the issues of alienation and violence among the members of our own social system. I strongly believe that we can construct such a discourse, drawing upon the ideas of historical materialism, modern communication theory, and the ideas of feminist scholarship from such thinkers as Marx,[2] Weinbaum,[3] and Wilden.[4]

Metascientific Analysis

I will begin with some of Wilden's ideas on the nature of what a new discourse of science should include. His concept of what a scientific discourse should not be is somewhat easier to understand than his statements on what it should be. According to Wilden: "Any scientific theory or position which looks like a metaphor of the dominant ideology of our society or which can be constructed as a contribution to psychological, social, and material alienation of any class or group in the world society must come under immediate suspicion. It must then be subjected to a metascientific and contextual evaluation before being accepted as valid or useful or truth."[4]

The key concepts we need to look at are metascientific and contextual evaluation. A metascientific analysis concerns itself with what a scientific discourse is saying within its methods about observation and analysis. That is, does the scientific statement have short-term usefulness or can it make a contribution to the general problem of human existence within a process of increasing alienation? Let us look at the metamessages of cultural relativism as espoused by the Boasian school of anthropology. In its early form it was a radical critique of assumed patterns of Western progress and a strongly stated and somewhat successful critique of the emerging scientific racism of the early 1900s. Within this context, the Boasian school has a legitimate claim to our praise; however, here is also where the problem emerges. In stressing the mental equality of all cultures, relativism put the economically poorer cultures in the political situation of having a symbolic system equal to any in the world, while the dominant cultures, which lacked such symbolic wealth but controlled the material wealth, were willing to accept all sorts of symbolic changes that did not affect their domination or materially enhance the supposedly symbolic rich cultures. Thus we now find ourselves trying to explain why such symbolically rich people find our material world more interesting than their cosmically rich cultures. The Boasian school gave people dignity through admiration of their cultures, but nothing to eat.

The metamessages of our own discourses and the reality of other people's existence become neutralized in the message networks of our own social system because of a lack of any contextual base to either our messages or descriptions. Thus, we need to recognize that people live in and react not to their culture or their society but to the overall context in which they find themselves. In fact, though we tend not to want to understand this, we in the areas of nursing and anthropology already deal with people in terms of contexts, which we forget when we attempt to analyze people's behavior in terms of our limited epistemology. However, we still need to define what we mean by a contextual analysis.

Labor, Time, and Space Considerations

There are three elements that have to be used in making a contextual study: *labor, time* and *space*. ***Labor*** *refers to the nature of people's ranges of productive activity in terms of age and gender.* That is, we wish to deal with how people maintain and continue their ways of life in terms of how they accumulate and distribute the general surplus that they produce through their labor activity. If a group is a foraging and hunting social unit, we would need to know who does what kind of labor in terms of gender and age, who produces the surplus in terms of labor role, who has access to both these labor roles and the surplus, and what is the nature of the power relationships associated with surplus accumulation. Also we would be concerned with knowing how people are treated and cared for in terms of their labor role and access to a general surplus within the system. These are relational questions that can tell us about the nature of labor within any form of productive activity from foraging to industrial capitalism.[3]

Time *refers to when the behavior we observed is taking place.* If we are concerned with understanding the nature of care among native Americans, we need to be explicit about whether we are talking about native Americans prior to European contact, during the period of contact, or as part of their enforced lives upon the reservation.

Space *refers to where such behaviors take place and under what kind of conditions.* There is a tremendous difference in the range of people's behaviors in terms of the spatial conditions in which they find themselves. The behavior of a group of horticulturalists will be different in terms of what time period we are dealing with and the nature of the spacial conditions available for such people. For example, the modern people of the Pacific are not the same people of 100 years ago or even 30 years ago. The history of modern capitalism and socialism has altered the nature of the labor of these people, thus altering both the nature of the time and space conditions. It is a curious procedure we use in the area of ethnography. We go into an area to describe the culture of a particular group of people, which generally means some picture of a traditional way of life. To do this, we have to ignore the actual conditions in which people are living and capture glimpses of what has been maintained of their past life. Then, after we have studied the traditional way of life and published that, we go back to study how they are coping because we have no point of comparison except a fallacious assumption about a traditional cultural past. Without the use of a contextual framework, we collect situational impressions of both the people we are studying and ourselves from the overall real context in which both ourselves and our informants are living. That is, we confuse logical levels when we encounter different social systems. Logical levels refer to the fact that some structures have dominance over others and that without such an arrangement certain structures could not exist.

Wilden suggested that the simplest test of how this could be understood is to ask which structures would survive if other structures were removed. Contrary to our own pronouncement, the structures of nature dominate over those of human structures. To Wilden, a simple test is that if you remove humans from nature it will continue to exist; however, if you remove nature, we cannot continue to exist. Thus, the structures of nature dominate over the general structures of humans. As Wilden observed, "The problem for us is not to save the environment, but to save our relationship to it."[4] Wilden was not suggesting patterns of determinism but that when we wish to account for particular structures we have to understand how each structure is related to others in a general system. And within that general system some structures are from a higher logical order than others. Furthermore, without addressing the question of contexts, we then miss the reality of the ordering of particular structures within the system we are looking at. Going back to the problem of looking at social systems without a contextual framework, we confuse the level of content and action. Ethnographically, we tend to describe a particular content in different social systems as if that content were a societal or cultural feature of the system we have been examining. What we tend to miss is the patterns of action that people have created or been forced to accept that lead towards the expression of the particular content that we have been labeling as their culture. Thus, when we discuss *curandismo,* we label all the content factors of this process as cultural and rarely address how it has come about that a large segment of the population in the American Southwest is either being forced out of or choosing not to use modern health care. It is this historical action that leads towards the behavioral patterns important to our concerns as health anthropologists, not the endless list of cures and rituals that are used by particular *curanderos.* This I will develop more fully later, for there are two other issues we have to address in order to understand the nature of the discourse we need to construct.

Three Levels of Meaning

When we look at the nature of our own discourse, or for that matter discourses of any group of people, we have to understand that they can and do take place at three levels of meaning: the real, the symbolic and the imaginary. How these three levels of meaning are ranked is a matter of the power relationships within a social system. How a discourse gets constructed, transmitted, received and the orderings of levels within that discourse are also a reflection of societal patterns of power. The real are those forms of communication that deal with the actualities of the dialectic relationship between one's self and the multiple contexts within which one lives; the symbolic deals with the probable forms of action that one can create to understand, alter, and transform the particular relationships within one's context, and the imaginary deals with those patterns of information and action that act to confuse the person as to what the real is and to weaken or neutralize one's symbolic actions down to nothing but empty symbols. The real for the urban poor of Oaxaca is the constant double bind of low income persons in a society that requires high cash resources to obtain any of its benefits—including health care. The symbolic deals with how people create strategies of survival and hope (which include concepts of health and caring) in terms of the real conditions that provide them with little in the way of encouragement. The imaginary involves total use of the super-structure of this system, primarily the areas of education and health that continually attempt to tell poor people that both their lack of income and the problems which result from a lack of income, particularly in the area of illness, represent their lack of understanding of how a system works. And if the poor would focus on how to better educate themselves, then they could reduce their problem. We tend to reinforce this imaginary analysis by stressing to those in power that they too need to better educate themselves on the reality of poverty, and we offer them explanatory concepts such as culture, society and personality. Because such concepts lack a contextual base in terms of ourselves and others, we then end up endorsing the most imaginary assumptions of all, namely that the problems of poverty, health and illness are just matters of education. The real and symbolic worlds of the urban poor get lost by such a discourse. This happens because we accept the rules of the powerful bourgeoisie which they themselves do not follow.

Let me explain this briefly. Science emerged in the Western world as part of a capitalist triumph over the feudal order. Capitalists claimed that their new world order would be one based upon rational analysis in opposition to the use of religious or spiritual information to control behavior within feudal systems. Science was thus required to create and maintain a level of objectivity so that it could be granted a domain of activity within that new world order based upon the growth of rationality and planning. Over the years the role of objectivity—which is basically an acceptance of a possibility of a negation of one's premises—emerged as the concept of value-free science. That is, somehow both ourselves as scientists and our works were not supposed to reflect our basic values and hopes. To participate in this new world order we were not allowed the basic element of our labor—the instrumental use of our own knowledge. If we wish to be scientists, we are then to do research without imposing our own values. After somebody else has used our knowledge, we can then react as citizens to how that knowledge has been used. This is a classic example of alienation. That is, we have and continue to be separated from the creation of our labor, the knowledge we produce as human scientists. In fact, the continued attraction that cultural and social anthropology has is that it gives an imaginary means of avoiding this process of alienation. We need to recognize that all forms of knowledge are, in fact, instrumental and we as scientists, nurses, and anthropologists have as much right and need to determine how knowledge is used, not as scientists nor as citizens, but as real persons. Thus, we need to be able to construct a definition of culture and caring in which the possible instrumental use of these terms can be directed toward a confrontation with processes of alienation within our own social system. I would like to suggest that the concept of praxis can be such a concept.

The history of the development of the anthropological concept of culture has been attempted by many, with little success in defining the process beyond the hope that it does exist in some fashion. The one work that I have found to rise above all this confusion is Bauman's book, *Culture as Praxis*.[5] The following will be an attempt to summarize Bauman's argument and to explore its use in understanding the process of caring. Bauman provided an extensive review of what the concept of culture was supposed to have meant in particular schools of thought (such as the difference between British and American anthropology in terms of the importance of culture) and how it has been misused. He showed that much of the confusion over the term *culture* arises from the attempt to place the process of cultural action within a closed scientific discourse requiring verification of a process that in fact transcends the limited techniques of verification embedded in positivistic science. Bauman contended that the process of culture deals with the formation of behavioral and symbolic ordering, which allows human beings to confront and transform the conditions in which they find themselves. In other words, humans order the world, not to make it permanent but to understand and transform it. This ordering is a collective effort through producing and reproducing meaning in terms of labor, time and space. To Bauman, the process of culture is analogous to the process of human praxis. ***Praxis** is the ability to impose order upon chaos;* this allows for collective human action for survival. More importantly, through ordering, humans are able to create meaningful actions that lead toward social change. Culture then becomes a dialectic process in which humans order their universe of action to allow for a meaningful existence.[5]

Content and Action

To illustrate, let us go back to the differences between content and action. It is not the form or content of human behavior that makes it consistent, but that we consistently act to make our lives meaningful and significant. We can do this through gaining control over what we create in the context in which we find ourselves. It is only through this power of ordering that we can alter our conditions. However, when we are asked to demonstrate or verify this field of action, we fall victim to the limited positivistic epistemology of counting. In accepting that meaning of behavior, we are forced to turn the dynamic processes of action into static elements of content. This produces a mundane and vulgar description of human behavior as a process of a constant adaptation to the real (survival), and we are always wondering how it is that people change. Furthermore, those who have laid down the dictates of positivism can clearly see the mundanity of our attempt and thus continue to monitor the level of the scientific import of our work. Thus, in accepting the dictates of an alienated form of inquiry, we lock ourselves into dead-ended conceptual frameworks and lose power to alter our own conditions and those of the people we seek to help.

The content of any particular cultural system is not very important to either the cultural system or to anyone attempting to understand the behavior and aid in the caring of other human beings. Content is the end product of human action directed towards ordering a domain of meaning in terms of the historical conditions that people find themselves in. Health anthropologists observe the content of people's history—such as the role of social networks and caring and the appointment of particular persons who perform rituals; then we extract that process from social context and label that process from social context and label it as the people's culture. We then go back ten years later, under new conditions and start labeling what we are witnessing as cultural change. In fact, what has changed is a multilevel process involving the rearrangement of the nature of people's labor use, thus placing people in different sets of space and time relationships. This rearrangement will necessitate a change in the ordering of people's lives so they can attempt to create new meanings for existence. When dealing with the onslaught of capitalism, many such creations will not work because the context no longer exists for there to be any meaningful behavior associated with the order (such as the ghost dance of native Americans). Some confrontations we identify are in fact short-term adaptations to difficult conditions, such as urban poverty or class domination; whereas others, such as the revolutionary activity of the Amazon Indians of Ecuador, are concrete attempts at the construction of meaningful behavior in the real context of the underdeveloped capitalism of Latin America. However, we tend to miss all the above processes because we are still back at the ethnographic laboratory labeling content as human behavior.

Bauman[5] suggested a way out of this conceptual double bind. He stressed that culture should be defined as a process of action which is a constant critique of any given reality. That is, culture is not the end product of some assumed historical process; it is the process of history itself. The wide array of ethnographic information we have collected under the label of cultural behavior is a strong endorsement for human creativity, and all the empirical proof that we need to demonstrate that we can understand both our own and other people's immediate conditions, perceive means to alter such conditions, and change social conditions. Culture is thus the constant critique of all the epistemologies of determinism ranging from social biology to materialism. In terms of this argument, we need to see that culture illustrates the domain of people's real and symbolic actions and provides us with a means to demystify the domain of the imaginary. This concept of culture provides us with a tool to fight against the processes that threaten both ourselves and the people we wish to care for; that is, we can talk seriously and concretely about how to transform the context of our own social alienation.

It seems to me that nurses and anthropologists have accepted Illich's general critique of the modern medical industry, and thus we wish to draw upon different social systems to build some kind of holistic health care system. We pull out particular contents of social systems that we think will aid in this endeavor. I think we are wrong. The existence of folk health care systems is not an endorsement for the practice of holistic health but a strong condemnation of the modern medical industry, whose very structure prevents it from providing health care for the total population that needs it. As to the pragmatic and curing powers of folk health care, they need to be studied and confirmed. But we must face the fact that many of these behaviors are short-term adaptations of people who have found themselves in situations where their worlds have become meaningless.

Culture as Process Reality

Let me give two examples of how we can look at *culture* as a process of a critique of existing reality. For this I will draw upon the works of some artists: the work of Nichols[6] on the Spanish-speakers of northern New Mexico and the art of *reggae* in Jamaica. Nichols' book is a long historical novel dealing with the living conditions of Chicanos in northern New Mexico. Though the author is an Anglo, his feeling for both the region and the people is powerful and accurate. The storyline involves a small mountain town that over the years has lost most of its productive land to corporate interests, with the remaining land now being threatened by a tourist park. The novel deals with how all the characters—though predominantly the Chicanos—confront what they have wanted out of their lives, what they have been able to attain in terms of the constraints upon their lives, and how they can change. The Chicanos come to grips with what their past and present have been, and the novel concludes with the Chicanos redefining what they are and what they have been. They achieve this, not through protecting their lifestyles in terms of a cultural system, but by organizing a struggle against those who were dominating them. To attain their victory, they have to redefine several decades of history and abandon many forms of behavior that outsiders had labeled as their culture. Though the book is fictional, its subject matter is quite real.

Reggae comes from the urban slums of Jamaica. It is music full of political, social, economic, and religious themes. It comes from a combination of the extreme conditions of urban and rural poverty and the religious movement of the *Rasta,* which is a back-to-Africa movement based on the images of Haile Selassie, Marcus Garvey, and the smoking of *ganja.* The major *reggae* artists have come from the slums, and their music expresses that background. They have defined a new language, religion, and politics in their music and use them to force changes in their present living conditions and those conditions which involve the future of their children. Their songs are not harsh or bitter, but openly political and revolutionary in their vision. They have organized their general views around the concept of dread. They define dread as an awareness of what the conditions they live under are, and what brought them about. It also contains within it a meaning or an awareness that change will come, they will be the ones to create the change, and that such changes will involve both new lives for themselves and also for the people who have been oppressing them. In fact, I would maintain the *reggae* concept of dread is the best metaphor we can have for the idea of culture as praxis.

Conclusion

Now, how does this epistemological argument refer back to the problem of caring? Nursing and anthropology share two important aspects: both disciplines deal with people in terms of the real context in which they live. Unfortunately, both disciplines have attempted to explain that context in terms of some cultural model. When we deal with people in their own social context, we move beyond the limited discourse of science, which attempts to find ways to justify alienation with the use of such split realities as culture and society. However, when we ourselves wish to explain what we do, we tend to have our work and our hopes neutralized. How do we get beyond the double bind of our own social system?

Answering such a question cannot be done in a single paper; the answers have to come from a collective confrontation within the disciplines of nursing and anthropology. First, we need to rethink the whole language we use in attempting to account for other people's behavior. If my argument about culture is correct, then related terms such as society, community, family, and personality also have to be rethought. If one of these terms is misleading, then they all are. We need to see that many of the problems we confront in our professions have little to do with other people's social systems. In providing care for these others, we need to recognize that perhaps the ones who need care are ourselves. Often the assumptions of cultural relativism hide the real problems of health and illness. Nurses and anthropologists find themselves concerned with the plight of the powerless people who are themselves attempting to lessen their domination. However, our main means of aid is to simply offer ethnic and cultural respect. Left unanswered is this question: Who are the powerless—other cultures, or our own powerlessness in relationship to the dominant others in our own social system? If we can respect the lives of other people, then do we not also attain some kind of respect from the dominant powers in our own social system? This paper has attempted to point out that such assumptions end up negative for both the people we wish to aid, and ourselves.

Acceptance of a split reality is acceptance of an alienated epistemology which assumes that meaning and significance are separate from people's daily lives. We continually use concepts that separate the subjective and objective domains of human behavior. They are not separate realities.

To conclude, let me suggest that we can use the concept of care as a part of the range of meaning meant by the idea of culture as praxis. Praxis is the constant and spontaneous creation of meaningful behavior in the lives of human beings. Culture is the historical context in which praxis takes place. Thus, culture is the human action of people making, defining, altering, and transforming the means which they have to attain meaning. To me, caring should be a health science that looks for the relations of human actions that can illustrate these processes and attempts, not to turn a particular context into an imaginary tool we think can be used to right our own powerlessness.

Caring has to be felt at the level of the real and the symbolic. We should fight against the neutralizing powers of the imaginary. We must create strategies of care that accept the existence of others but refuse to allow them the status of dominant other.

References

1. Krader L: The Dialectic of Civil Society. Netherlands, Van Gorcum, 1976.
2. Marx K: Capital, Vol I. New York, International Press, 1967.
3. Weinbaum B: The Curious Courtship of Women's Liberation and Socialism. Boston, South End Press, 1978.
4. Wilden A: System and Structure. London, Tavistock, 1972.
5. Bauman Z: Culture as Praxis. London, Routledge & Kegan Paul, 1973.
6. Nichols J: The Milagro Beanfield War. New York, Random House, 1978.

Cross-Cultural Hypothetical Functions of Caring and Nursing Care

9

Madeleine Leininger, R.N., Ph.D., Lh.D., F.A.A.N.

Purpose

The purpose of this paper is to present some hypothetical and universal functions of caring as a heuristic approach to advance the science and humanistic dimensions of caring. In this paper I also offer a multilevel model to study cross-cultural caring and nursing care functions and practices along with some general premises and theoretical statements to guide future investigations on caring.

The Need for Cross-Cultural Study of the Functions of Caring

With any discipline or profession, its members have the responsibility to conceptualize and implement their knowledge and skills for a particular society, and contribute to the knowledge of the world at large. Disciplines exist to be generators of knowledge, and then if they are a profession, there is a responsibility to use the knowledge to serve humankind in professional ways. These aspects should be kept in mind in order to maintain both a discipline and professional status. In the future, it will also be important to maintain a cross-cultural focus of professional knowledge domains.

In the nursing and health disciplines, a cross-cultural focus is needed to gain insight and explain health-illness caring and curing from cultural viewpoints. Cross-cultural theories and research related to caring are extremely important today, and will be more so in the future. Caring attitudes and behaviors will be important to maintain peace, communication, and daily working roles in any culture. More caring and less war threats are needed for future international health living modes. The transcultural nursing subfield is in a unique position to advance such a perspective. This leads to my presentation of some transcultural hypotheses about the function of caring in human cultures, and with thought to human relatedness and nursing care metatheories, research, and practice aspects.

The first major hypothesis is that ***cross-cultural caring*** and ***care functions*** *are critical factors for human growth, self and group actualization, human development, and survival for human cultures* throughout the long history of humankind.[1] This hypotheses is important for the cross-cultural examination of the universal function of caring. This function appears to be logical, real, and symbolical when one considers that *Homo sapiens* has existed in this world for more than one million years, and in very precarious environments. The ability of humans to care for themselves and each other through time must have been a critical factor for survival of all human cultures. Humans must have been attentive to and involved in helping the very young offspring, the handicapped, injured, or sick to have led to human wellbeing and their survival today. What other human act or behavior could have been more vital to the human race than caring for self and others amid diverse circumstances and highly unpredictable social and physical environments?

In the past, natural and humanmade disasters must have called for a quality of human relatedness, protection, nurturance, and assistance under stressful and unknown conditions. Anthropologically speaking, human compassion and concern for others through caring was not only essential to preserve and maintain the human race, but to retain and develop human cultures through time. Human groups must have realized that no society or culture could have existed or maintained themselves without reciprocal caring relationships. Helping people in time of need and helping groups to achieve their daily living needs appears to be the essence of caring.

The second major function of cross-cultural caring flows from the first. I believe ***caring activities, behaviors,*** *and* ***processes*** *linked human groups together in a sense of mutual interdependence and interrelatedness* in order to achieve desired human tasks, maintain health, and to survive. This function also appears logical and self-evident for cultures to survive through time, and has some suggested support from the anthropological literature. However, it has not been specifically discussed in relation to health and wellness behaviors. Such a major function leads to other hypotheses such as: 1) The more signs of caring, the greater the signs of interdependence or mutual interrelatedness among groups; 2) The greater the evidence of beneficial care, the more evident that individuals are able to perform their goals and contributions to a community.

Caring appears to be a universal function to link people together through relationships between caregivers and care receivers. The caregiver's role in most cultures is to provide helpful acts. Reciprocal supportive measures to others should have enabled people to meet daily living and crisis conditions. The role of caregivers to help other human beings with obvious needs or to anticipate their needs, must have been an important societal function, but it also helped to link individuals and groups together in a sense of interdependence. One could also conjecture that linkage attitudes of caring behavior helped to prevent feuds, crimes, destructive behaviors, and some forms of social deviance in a society. At the same time, human satisfactions through caring linkages must have increased trust, empathy, and sociopolitical ties. Thus, caring not only helped to link people together, but it also helped to promote a sense of responsibility for one another. Linkage with mutual interdependence of helping and sharing with each other must have been a major function of caring for people in the past as it is today.

A third hypothetical function of cross-cultural caring is that ***caring*** *played an important role in protecting and maintaining humans* who were ill or under the threat of illness, as well as helping people who were suffering from accidents, fatal diseases, or a community malaise. Humans have always had some type of health care, whether from professional or folk care providers. What forms of health-illness care existed in the past? How did caring behaviors protect individuals from illness, death, maintain wellness, or help individuals recover from an illness state? Protective, nurturant, and assistive functions of caring must have been essential to maintain the human race over millions of years. Such protective and maintenance caring behaviors would have been learned from caregivers and then transmitted to other caregivers in future generations. Cultural transmission through enculturation processes related to caring behaviors appears essential to human groups. Forms of artistic, humanistic and scientific modes of caring would have been evident in the past, but they remain limitedly known in professional health systems today. While the nursing profession has laid claim to giving nursing care, or providing care to others, for more than a century, still the specific scientific and humanistic knowledge base and form of care remains virtually unknown, along with the specific caring skills, their meaning and functions.[2]

Some other questions need to be asked: If caring activities and attributes were not present in a life-threatening illness or accident situation, what were the chances for human survival in the past? When people were dying, did caring attitudes and activities make a difference in the final outcome? In nursing, we believe therapeutic care makes a difference, but the how and why of such care is often obscure. Nurses, too, know by experience that if good nursing care is not available or is withdrawn, the client soon dies. As nurses, we believe that therapeutic caring attitudes and activities play an important role in maintaining wellness, preventing death, and making dying more acceptable or comfortable. These cross-cultural or universal functions of nursing as professional caring remain areas for future verification. Moreover, the specific functions and relationships of care to culture and society have only recently been explored by a few nurse researchers.

A fourth major function of caring is that ***caring behaviors, activities*** *and* ***processes*** *serve society to help prevent aspects of human misery, reality stresses, and socially disruptive conditions,* and these functions are culturally based and institutionalized. If such caring attitudes and activities were not institutionalized in a culture or society, one would predict socially disruptive behaviors and chaotic situations. The reason is that human beings are never completely independent or isolated in life. Instead, people are social and cultural beings linked to each other. People frequently face crises, problems, and frustrations in relationship to other individuals, due to changing social, political, and economic conditons. Caring, I contend, is a cultural mechanism or safety valve that helps to alleviate mass suicides, homocides, and other societal deviancy problems. Helping individuals, families, and groups with human life problems such as famine, floods, earthquakes, mass accidents, and other catastrophies as well as economic and political repressive conditions, all necessitate that caring be institutionalized and serve as a cultural mechanism in societies.

Caring is a response to helping the helpless in times of need. Caring acts and behaviors appear to be essential to sustain a helpless individual, society, or culture. What would happen to a society if caring acts were not present to deal with the many societal stresses and problems? Without care, there would probably be mass chaos. Recent occurrences of natural- and human-made catastrophies in the world reflect the need for caring attitudes and behaviors as an imperative for human survival and protection. During disasters, I have often seen a spirit of helpfulness (or caring) prevail, to help alleviate human misery and the pain of great loss. I have heard people say: "Those caring folks helped me to live on, rebuild my home, and try to start anew in a nearby area." Therefore, I believe caring has long been an essential cultural value to help people maintain societies and to help alleviate human misery, face reality stresses, and deal with common human conditions. The need to identify caring modes and mechanisms, as well as the functions and variations among different individuals, social institutions, and cultures seems imperative for a full understanding of caring in human loving contexts, and during illness and wellness states.

The fifth major function of **cross-cultural caring** *is to promote and sustain human qualities and attributes of people.* Without caring attitudes, it is possible that people would act more like animals or non-hominids. Caring attributes, such as maintaining interest in other humans, showing concern for the welfare of others, tending to the special needs of people, protecting them from danger or harm, and being compassionate and thoughtful—all seem important and desired features of being human.[2] In fact, when such attributes are not evident, one often hears such comments as, "He/she is like a wild animal," or, "There's no humanness in him/her." The feelings of concern, empathy, thoughtfulness, and helpfulness to other humans appear to be extremely important qualities of being human. Persons with noncaring attitudes might be viewed as those who are indifferent to others, show no signs of compassion or concern, and who are selfish and without thought for other human needs and life conditions. In some cultures, to be caring is to be more Christ-like, or to have the sacred qualities of a special human being. In other cultures, caring is reflected with protection, tenderness, and other attributes. Studies are needed to examine past and current ideas of noncaring and caring persons and how these values are related to human qualities. We need to address these questions: Do noncaring persons become destructive to self and others more readily than caring persons? Are crime, homocide, and other social problems symptomatic of noncaring humans? How can one change noncaring to caring behavior to make people more humane?

The sixth major function of **cross-cultural caring** *is to facilitate curing* *modalities in health and non-health situations.* Since I contend that there can be no curing without caring, then this proposition leads to the idea that caring is essential and must be present for curing to occur.[2] Caring attitudes, processes, and activities support curing modalities. The relationship of caring to curing appears close; however, I believe we must know more about caring to understand curing. From my 30 years of clinical caring and observations with clients, I find that while physicians do some therapeutic curative work on clients through surgery and other medical modes, without therapeutic nursing care, clients will die or have a difficult recovery. Therefore, it appears to me that *caring* activities and attitudes, with all its subtle aspects, are essential for clients to recover from surgery, medications, and curing regimes. Descriptive caring documentation and other validation is often not presented by nurses, and so *curing* is often viewed as *the* therapeutic or scientific medium, or the explanation for recovery. Caring processes and patterns generally fail to get recognition as the recovery factor because of the overriding professional emphasis on physicians' curing modes. In a way, it is like women not getting recognition for their important roles in socializing, maintaining the home, and child care practices. How caring helps clients by different nursing interventions needs visibility, with research documentation, and especially, how *caring* is essential to any *curing.*

Although there are other cross-cultural functions, these six major functions can stimulate nurses to think about the body of knowledge yet to be discovered and tested about caring phenomenon. Currently caring remains not only limitedly studied, but the most devalued, obscure, mystical (and mythical) aspect of human health services. The economic rewards and social sanctions for care are also miniscule in the United States and in other countries. Professional women as caregivers are neglected for their caring roles. Hence, much work lies ahead in the development of the uncut gem which is the key to human relatedness, growth, protectiveness, recovery, and survival.

Multilevel Conceptual Model for Caring

For further study of the phenomenon of caring, I offer a multilevel structural model to conceptualize and analyze the scope, nature, and structures of caring phenomenon (see Figure 9.1). In the model below, one can visualize several different levels and areas to study the caring activities and functions of the individual, family, system, cultural, societal, and world levels.

In studying these different caring levels, descriptive data of patterned caring processes, functions, and behaviors of caring are needed as well as the outcomes of caring to the individual, family, and society. Levels A and B require the highest level of abstractions, and are the broadest views of caring. They offer many theoretical possibilities and create more explanatory power than the lower levels of E and F. Some of the above predictions I have made about the cross-cultural *functions* of caring were examples of high-level abstractions. With level C, one would study specific cultures such as the Anglo-

FIGURE 9.1

A MULTILEVEL STRUCTURAL CARING MODEL

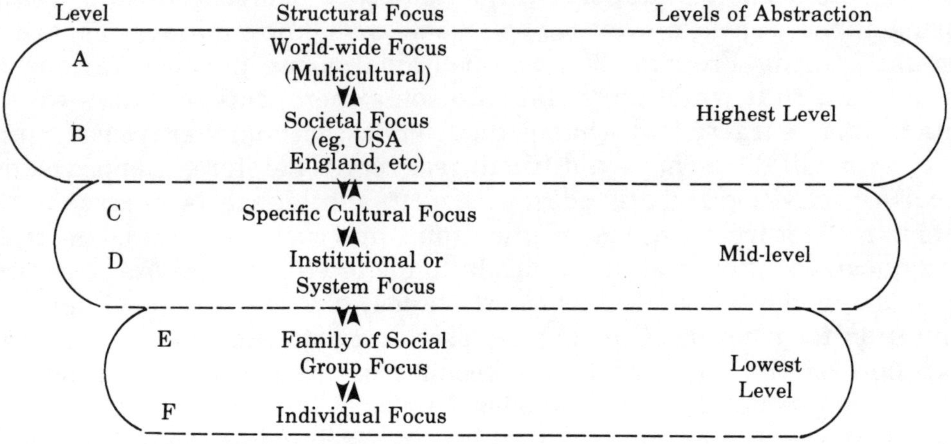

American, Mexican-American, and others, to identify how caring is structured within the culture and its particular functions in serving the people. This is the level in which I have been studying and classifying 30 cultures regarding cross-cultural caring patterns and processes as well as caregiver and care recipient behaviors. (Unpublished research from *A Taxonomy of Transcultural Caring and Nursing Care Behaviors)*. Findings from this level would ultimately contribute to levels A and B and should be reflected in levels D, E, and F through specific empirical data.

Level D reflects the institutional or system level of analysis and would include a study of caring in social institutions and such systems as education, legal, political, economic, and kinship. Caring behaviors and patterns of philosophical and manifest behaviors would be examined. The role of expectations, values, norms of institutions, and systems would be examined at level D. With levels E and F, one would study and analyze families, social groups, and individuals with respect to caring structuring, functions, and processes. The concrete or emprical manifestations of caring would also be documented. These levels are much more familiar to nurses than the abstract levels of A, B, C, and D. Specific care activities (or the absence of care) to an individual or family member within the home or health institutions could be studied at levels E and F, and could be linked to show relationships with the levels A, B, C, and D. Nurses prepared in anthropology and sociology could help nurses and others to examine the higher levels of analysis in A, B, and C. The interplay and interrelationships among *all* levels of the model are important for a complete analysis of caring. The use of this model as a conceptual, research, and analytical tool has many advantages to assure the full explication of caring knowledge, eg, structure, function, and process. Presently, nursing knowledge about caring is at levels A and B, and some of this knowledge is vague or imprecise.

Humanistic and Scientific Caring

Since most health professionals today tend to believe that anything labeled "scientific" is "objective" and "truthful in nature", it is important to consider what Higgins mentioned in the previous chapter, and what other researchers have said, and reflect upon the functional and historical reasons for the rise of the scientific method, and particularly the neglected humanistic, subjective, and covert dimensions of human behavior.[3] For heuristic and analytical purposes, we should to differentiate between humanistic and scientific caring in order to identify the characteristics of each aspect or focus of caring.[1] It appears to me that the humanistic aspects of care tend to be devalued and deemphasized with current overemphasis on technological care activities in the United States.

For clarity, I define ***humanistic caring*** *as the subjective feelings, experiences, and interactional behaviors between two or more persons (or groups)* in which assistive or enabling acts are performed generally without prior sets of verified or tested knowledge. Often humanistic caring is manifest by warm and thoughtful interpersonal verbal and non-verbal responses to another individual or group. In contrast, ***scientific caring*** *refers to those tested activities and judgments in assisting an individual or group,* based upon verified and quantified knowledge related to specific variables. Often, scientific caring is reflected in the precise use of technological instruments, the use of diagnostic words and acts, and in explicit and empirically known physical care activities. In time, we should blend the humanistic and scientific aspects, but we must first know what we are blending or uniting together. Humanistic care must be given as much attention as the scientific aspects, and considerably more attention than technical and physical care.

Premises to Guide Future Cross-Cultural Caring Investigations

Below are some premises, key questions, and theoretical statements to guide future studies in cross-cultural caring studies. They can be stated as follows:[2,4,5]

1) Caring activities, processes, and attitudes are essential to help maintain wellness and to prevent illness, disabilities, and handicaps in individuals, families, and cultural groups.
2) Every culture has caring modalities expressed through their institutions that help maintain and sustain human attributes and prevent social disruption and unfavorable human conditions.
3) Cross-cultural expressions of human caring differ in form, functions,

processes, and activities; however, there are some identifiable universal features among them.

4) Why is caring not economically valued and financially rewarded in the Unites States?
5) What is universal about caring behaviors, processes, and activities among all human cultures?
6) Why has caring not been rigorously addressed until recently as a generic concept of nursing care?
7) Are humanistic caring attributes peculiar to women professional and nonprofessional caregivers?
8) What are the essential criteria for being a professional care-provider?
9) What is distinctive about nursing as a caring profession?

There is a great potential for many disciplines to study caring phenomenon, but especially for the nursing profession if it wishes to make caring one of the distinctive features of the discipline. As nursing research studies and findings increase, efforts must be made to communicate professional caring to the public, so that recognition and rewards will be forthcoming to nursing for its contributions to society. Research monies are also greatly needed to study a long neglected area of human health services. Many of the questions identified in this paper need to be studied to develop a *science of caring* and *humanistic caring knowledge.* In the meantime, my optimism remains, as well as my belief that caring is one of the most crucial and important concepts yet to be discovered about human behavior and health care services. Furthermore, I hold that caring is not only the essence of nursing, but that it is essential for *all* human and health services in the professional and non-professional world.

References

1. Leininger M: Humanistic Care: An Alive, Dormant, or Lost Art? Read at the Seventh Annual Maryam Smith Memorial Lecture, University of Utah, Salt Lake City, Utah, May 24, 1973.
2. Leininger, M: The Phenomenon of Caring. American Nurses' Foundation (Nursing Research Report), Vol 12, No 1, February, 1977.
3. Leininger M: Transcultural Nursing Research Program. Paper presented for Kappa Chapter, Sigma Theta Tau, Catholic University of America, April 12, 1980.
4. Leininger M: Transcultural Nursing: Concepts, Theories and Practices. Chapters 1 and 2. New York: John Wiley & Sons, 1978.
5. Leininger M: Cross-Cultural Caring: Theories and Practices. In preparation for publication in 1981.

The Interrelatedness of the Caring Patterns in Black Children and Caring Process Within Black Families

10

Barbara Guthrie, R.N., M.S.N.

Overview

The purpose of this research project is to describe a theory of caring from the perspective of human science nursing. The author recognizes that many theories of caring are emerging. The specific focus of this project is the interrelatedness of caring patterns of black children and caring process within black families.

An overview of human science nursing in the form of assumptions about man, family, caring, and health will provide a basis for the theoretical framework which provided the underpinnings for the descriptive method utilized in the pilot study. A sample of the pilot study results is discussed with implications for nursing theory, practice, and research.

Introduction

This research project describes the interrelatedness of caring patterns of black children and the family process of caring from a human science nursing perspective. Human science nursing theory is emerging within the current scientific revolution in nursing. Kuhn observed that "a scientific revolution is a transformation of a scientific image."[1] Human science nursing theory is the beginning of a new scientific image for nursing as it emerges toward the status of a scholarly discipline.

Parse,[2] author of the emerging theory of human nursing, describes the major concepts of man* and health which give rise to the fundamental subconcepts of the theory. The theory of human science nursing is generated from a synthesis of selected concepts from general system theory and existential phenomenology. The postulates derived from this conceptual framework further describe man and health in relationship to family, and they provide the basis for understanding caring in light of human science nursing theory.

One postulate that specifically exemplifies the theory and describes man is, "Man is an open synergistic being whose coexistence is a rhythmical pattern of interrelating with the environment."[2] This means that man and environment are recipro-

No distinction is made with respect to gender in this paper.

cally related. The reciprocity between man and environment means that there is a mutual and simultaneous exchange of energy which can be likened to an undulating wave. In the betweeness of man and environment, there is an ever increasing complexity in the nature of the undulating wave of energy which shows itself in man's rhythmical pattern of coexisting.†

Coexistence means that man's existence is always in relation with others. One dimension of the multi-faceted patterns of coexistence is the way man lives in his cultural heritage. Man's culture is a negentropic unfolding that is lived in the rhythmically changing situational context man cocreates with others. This rhythmical connectedness shows itself through patterns of expressions which are cocreated in the context of family. As members live in the contextual situation of family, the patterns of expression illuminate each member's wholeness.

Family, in light of human science nursing, is a way of being with another; this way of being with another is grounded in the desire to cooperate and please. The way a family lives and desires to cooperate and please is synergistic in that there is a working together through the synchrony of energy exchange in the betweenness. This synchronous energy exchange enhances family growing. As the family grows together it lives related in the cadence of separating and connecting, and through illumination of this cadence, ways of caring unfold.

Caring is the openness to subjectively experience the other's becoming. It means investing in another's life without focusing on return investment, having time to listen, and bearing witness to another's suffering and joy. It means putting one's self in the other's place, risking criticism for supporting another, risking the sharing of different perspectives, and having time to dwell with self as a means of self commitment in the context of family. The human science way of caring is expressed through man's living anger, pain, sadness, joy, and suffering, in situations with another. Through these dimensions of caring, the family senses are energized; that is, the family is able to transcend what is and move toward possibilities. In this emerging process of transcending, the family does not become embedded in the limits of the situation, but rather evolves toward different limits. As the family evolves through the changing meanings of family, it cocreates family health. Family health is the intersubjective process cocreated in the betweenness of family members which simultaneously enables and limits the family's ways of caring.[2] The preceding description of man, family caring, and health has provided the foundation for the focus of this research project.

Theoretical Framework

Parse's work on human science nursing provides the theoretical framework for this nursing research project. A synthetic statement extrapolated from the postulates by Parse[2] on health will be empirically tested in order to uncover the

---

†*For a partial definition of terms, see Chapter 13.*

interrelatedness of caring patterns and the family caring process. Family health is an open intersubjective process of being and becoming as experienced by the individual in the context of family's rhythmical coconstituting the process of transcending toward the possible. This negentropic unfolding of family health is lived through the patterns of expressing value priorities in situation. The delineation of value priorities reflects the family's freedom to choose in situations and bear responsibility for decisions which paradoxically enable and limit family health. The investigator's way of supporting families to enable them to synchronize energies towards change help to mobilize family possibilities in promoting growth.

Consistent with nursing perspectives, a theoretical framework for caring and language was developed from the works of Heidegger, Earner, Kempler, Leonard, Stetson, and Watzlawick. As Heidegger described the process of caring: "to be with another is to care."[3] He stated that everything one does can be understood as a way of caring, and that man's caring is lived through language.

Kempler[4] implicity spoke about caring when he stated the premise that all men are basically good and that they have a desire to cooperate and please in the context of rhythmical relatedness with others. Leonard,[5] also addressed rhythmical relatedness in this metaphor of human existence as a musical melody in life as man participates in dancing to the melody in a to-and-fro movement. Leonard continued by saying that when two beings are in the same field their waves of energy exchange, are in tune, and they experience a sense of connectedness. These waves of energy exchange, Leonard suggested, are the key to the creation of language. He further contended that language patterns differ from family to family. However, the rhythmical process of dancing to-and-fro is always there, echoing the essential connectedness that defines each family process as unique.

In *Pragmatics of Human Communication,* Watzlawick[6] looked at the relatedness of man from a systems perspective. He described openness in human interrelating as the exchange of energy and this exchange of energy as patterns of interaction. Watzlawick contended that, "man cannot communicate." Watzlawick implied that one's presence *is* participation. This participation communicates through patterns of expression which include movement, speaking, and silence through which a message value is exchanged with another which defines the relationship. For Watzlawick the creation of patterns of interaction reflect a specific behavior. The patterns of interactions are structured in the form of *content* and *relationships.* He described content as information sent, while relationship refers to the way the message is sent. Content and relationship together define the meaning of the interaction. Watzlawick described two rhythmical patterns of relating as symmetrical and complementary. Symmetrical is described as a pattern of languaging which reflects being in an equal position with another. There is a sense of mirroring which leads to a reciprocal confirmation. Complementary is a pattern of language which focuses on unequal positions. Watzlawick refers to this as, "one up, one down." This emphasizes the interlocking nature of the relationship which anticipates the other while at the same time providing reasons for the behavior of the other. These patterns of language relatedness evolve out of the betweenness of the process. These language patterns illuminate the what and how of being in relation with another.

Finally, Earner has brought the dimension of silence to language. She states the "silent dwelling is the wellspring of communication."[7] That is, in the listening, one is present to the other. This enables one to go beyond words to what is more than words.

In summary, this theoretical framework provided the basis for how family health is cocreated in the betweenness of family members and how the process of caring reflects living family health. It has been demonstrated that one of the profiles of caring which illuminates family health is the family member's patterns of language. These patterns of language are rhythmical in nature and relate to how one experiences his relatedness with another.

Method

Ethnocultural heritage of the sample included 20 black eighth-grade students and their predominantly Roman Catholic families. Video-taping equipment was used as a means to analyze the caring patterns of the children in their peer group and in their respective families. Both process and content were analyzed relative to the interactional patterns of students with their peer groups and their respective families. The purpose of this way of analyzing this data was to uncover how caring patterns in the individual families are stated in a peer relationship. The investigator, being an active observer in this project, did a content analysis of languaging as a caring pattern.

Pilot Study Results

The content analysis of one student and family uncovered the similarity of language patterns of caring from family process to peer group process. A specific situation will serve to explicate this finding. The subject expressed his way of caring for his peers through joking. It was noted that his joking prevailed especially when he anticipated a "put down" from a peer. This languaging of caring through a pattern of joking enabled the student to assume a complementary position with his peers. When this pattern of being with his classmates was illuminated for the student, he explained that in anticipation of being hurt, he makes a joke to prevent the pain. The investigator moved to reframe his joking as a way of caring for his peers in situations. This ultimately helped him to examine his way of being and move toward other possibilities. This same subject's languaging pattern of caring was observed in the context of his family of origin. The family was composed of the subject and his mother. Throughout the investigator's participation with this family, a similar pattern of languaging emerged between the mother and subject. It was noted that when a serious issue was being discussed, either mother or son would interject a joke as a means of lightening the seriousness of the issue. The mother promoted the subject's continuing pattern of joking through joining him in making jokes. The investigator, sensing the uncomfortableness of this joking pattern about serious issues, shared this perception with the family. Through reframing the mother and son's way of expressing caring through joking, the investigator moved to have the son and the mother negotiate when they wanted the other to be serious. Through much struggling, the investigator mobilized the two to synchronize their energies toward a different way of being together. What the mother requested from her son was that he refrain from making jokes at school. The son requested that his mother stop making jokes about his way of being with her and others.,

Evaluation

On a subsequent interaction with this subject in his peer group, the investigator noted that there was a noticeable change in the frequency of his joking patterns with them. Through talking with the subject's mother she noted that her son's joking in school had decreased. The subject also stated that his mother was beginning "to be with me in a more serious way."

Implications for Theory, Practice, and Research Development

The findings of this research project supported Parse's[2] human science theory of nursing by demonstrating that rhythmical participation is lived through languaging patterns of caring. As the nurse lives this theory in nursing practice, she broadens the scope of practice by attending to caring patterns as they emerge from family process. Furthermore, this study contributes to research through expanding the concept of family health through analysis of patterns of caring in a variety of ethnic cultural families.

References

1. Kuhn R: The Structure of Scientific Revolution. Chicago, Chicago Press, 1970, p 6.
2. Parse, RR: Human Science Nursing Postulates, copyright 1978 from the book Human Science Nursing Theory, in process.
3. Heidegger M: Being and Time. New York, Harper and Row, 1962, chapters 4 and 5.
4. Kempler W: Principles of Gestalt Family Therapy. Norway, AS Nodales Trykkert, 1974.
5. Leonard G: The Silent Pulse. New York, EB Dutton, 1978, p 23.
6. Watzlawick P: Pragmatics of Communication. New York: WW Norton, 1967, p 48, 51, 57.
7. Earner M: Silent Dwelling. Well Spring of Communication, Humanities XI, No 2, May 1975, pp 167-174.

Patients' and Staff Nurses' Perceptions of Supportive Nursing Behaviors: A Preliminary Analysis

Kathryn G. Gardner, R.N., M.S.
Erlinda Wheeler, R.N., M.S.

11

Nurses have long assumed that giving support to patients is an essential part of their practice. It is an assumption which has attracted little scientific attention. The meaning, operational definition, and consequences of support in nursing have yet to be determined.

A pilot study was designed to elicit nurses' and patients' perceptions of supportive nursing behaviors. The study was conducted in a regional medical center in the Northeast and utilized three inpatient specialty areas: surgery, medicine, and psychiatry. The study had three specific goals: 1) to determine which supportive nursing behaviors were perceived by nurses and patients as being most important; 2) to determine the overall extent of agreement or disagreement between the nurses' and patients' perceptions of supportive nursing behavior; and 3) to determine variation in the extent of agreement or disagreement between the nurses' and patients' perceptions of supportive nursing behaviors in each of the specialty areas of surgery, medicine, and psychiatry.

Method

A structured interview and a questionnaire were used in this study. The questionnaire is at the pilot stage of development and, therefore, has only face validity at this time. This paper summarizes the preliminary analysis of the questionnaire.

The questionnaire listed 67 behaviors previously described in nursing literature as supportive. These behaviors included physical, social, emotional, and cognitive activities of the nurse. A summary of the nursing literature on support has been described elsewhere.[1] Subjects were asked to rate each behavior on a seven-point Likert scale, ranging from absolutely important to not at all important. Patient and nurse subjects were given the same list of behaviors, but minor alterations in words were used to insure understanding by the patient subjects. The words used in the list of behaviors given to the patient subjects were not above the ninth-grade level of understanding. Patient subjects were asked to rate each nursing behavior according to how important they perceived the behavior was to the support of the patients. Nurse subjects were asked to rate each nursing behavior according to how important they perceived the behavior was in giving support to patients.

Trained research assistants administered the questionnaire and structured interviews to both nurse and patient subjects who volunteered to participate in the study. Confidentiality was assured by using code numbers, and privacy was provided by closing the door of the patient subject rooms or drawing the curtain around the patient if there were two patients in the room. Nurse subjects were interviewed separately and in a private room. Research assistants stayed with the subjects while they were interviewed and completed the questionnaire.

Sample

There were 74 nurse subjects who participated in the study: 21.6% of the subjects were from surgery, 43.2% from medicine, and 35.1% from psychiatry. The age range of the nurses was between 21 and 56 years, with over 74% of the sample younger than 33 years. The distribution of educational preparation of the nurse subjects was as follows: Diploma—22%; Associate's degree—26%; B.S. and above—52%. Differences in education between the specialty areas were not statistically significant, using chi square. Eighteen percent of the sample had worked less than one year in nursing. Forty percent had worked from one to four years, and the remaining 42% had worked more than four years.

There were 119 patients who participated in the study. Twenty-five percent of the patients were from surgery, 50% were from medicine, and 25% were from psychiatry. Age range of the patients was from 18 to 86 years, and 40% of the study population were between 46 and 55 years. The distribution of educational background of the patient subjects was as follows: 20% of the patients had not completed a high school education level, 36% were high school graduates, and the remaining 44% had more than a high school education. Differences in education between the specialty areas were statistically significant ($p < .05$), using chi square. More medical and surgical patients were educated beyond the high school level than psychiatric patients. Psychiatric patients had more patients with less than a high school education.

There were 57 men and 59 women, with the male population being over-represented (84%) in surgery and under-represented (33%) in psychiatry ($p < .05$). Patients in medicine were almost equally divided between males and females. Three patient subjects were not identified according to sex. The higher proportion of male patients in surgery was unexplainable and was considered a sampling error, since it is not typical of the overall population of surgical patients within the Medical Center. In psychiatry the relatively low proportion of male patients approximates the overall proportion of males in the psychiatric units within the Medical Center.

At the time patients participated in the study, their hospital stay ranged from 2 to 35 days with two patients being in the hospital for 2 days. When interviewed, 47% of the patient subjects were in the hospital for one week or less, 29% for less than two weeks, and 15% were in the hospital two weeks or more.

Results and Analysis of Data

The relative importance of each of the behaviors to each subject was ascertained by the following procedure. For each subject mean and standard deviation of their evaluation of the 67 behaviors was determined. For each individual the distribution across the 67 behaviors was transformed to one with a mean of 10 and a standard deviation of one. The result is a measure of the relative importance of each behavior as compared with the importance given by the same subject to other behaviors. A score of 10 shows that the behavior was assigned average importance, a score of nine shows one standard deviation below the average. The procedure adjusted for the possibility of differential response set between subjects as well as possible differences in the average absolute importance attributed to the 67 behaviors by the subjects.

A two-way analysis of co-variance across specialty areas and education with age as co-variate was done for the items rated by the nurse subjects; and a three-way analysis of co-variance across the specialty areas, education, and sex with age as the co-variate was done for the items rated by the patient subjects. The three-way analysis of co-variance for patients was carried out because patients were both males and females while nurses were almost all females. For this report, while the means are adjusted for age, education, and sex (for the patients), further analysis of these three variables will be ignored in order to concentrate on the effects of the specialty areas and the differences between nurses and patients.

The three nursing behavior items ranked by nurses in descending order of importance were: 1) show interest in patients; 2) create an environment where a patient feels free to express feelings; 3) take time to listen to patients. There was no statistically significant effect across specialty areas on the relative importance of the three most important supportive nursing behaviors as ranked by the nurses. The three items ranked as most important by the patients in descending order of importance were: 1) nurse helped me to feel confident that adequate care was provided; 2) nurse was friendly; 3) nurse showed interest in me. The first ten items ranked by nurses and patients were compared; three items appeared in both nurses' and patients' rankings of the first ten items. These items were: 1) show interest in patient; 2) assess patient; 3) provide moral support. There was no statistical difference in the three items across specialty areas.

Twenty-seven items were statistically significant ($p < .05$) between nurses' and patients' rankings of supportive behaviors. Out of these 27 items, 18 were statistically significant at the $p < .025$ level. Patients ranked the following items higher than nurses: 1) being friendly; 2) helping me to be calm by giving reassurance; 3) restore confidence; 4) provide physical care on time; 5) helping me not to feel alone. Nurses ranked the following items higher than patients: 1) listening to patients' feelings; 2) taking time to listen; 3) fostering family communication; 4) helping to establish realistic goals; 5) helping patients maintain personal integrity.

Sixteen items were perceived by patients as statistically significant ($p < .05$) across specialty areas: surgery, medicine, and psychiatry. Providing patients with moral support was perceived as relatively more important by psychiatric patients than medical and surgical patients. The nurses sharing feelings and thoughts, assisting them to gain control over their behavior, and helping them to solve their problems was perceived as relatively more important by psychiatric patients than medical and surgical patients. Nurses responding to patients' attempts at friendship was perceived as most important by medical patients and least important by surgical patients. Nine out of 13 physical care items in the questionnaire were ranked lower by psychiatric patients than by medical or surgical patients. Providing physical care on time and keeping the patient clean was perceived as relatively more important by medical patients than by surgical patients. Surgical patients perceived receiving physical comfort activities as relatively more important than medical patients did. Assisting the patient in maintaining comfortable body position was perceived as equally important by surgical and medical patients. In contrast to patients, only two items were perceived by nurses as statistically significant ($p < .05$) across specialty areas. These items were: 1) point out reality to patient; 2) stay with patient when he is upset.

Conclusion

For nurses in medical, surgical, and psychiatric areas, the relative importance of these 67 behaviors for supportive care was usually not affected by specialty area. In contrast, for patients in the three specialty areas the relative importance of the 67 behaviors varied by specialty for 16 items or 24% of the supportive nursing behaviors listed in the questionnaire.

There was no statistical significance between patients and nurses in their perceptions of supportive nursing behaviors for 40 behaviors, or 65% of the behaviors listed in the questionnaire. Both nurses and patients agreed that showing interest in the patient, assessing the patient, and providing moral support were among those behaviors most important to providing supportive care.

Patients and nurses disagreed to a statistically significant extent on the relative importance they assigned to 27 items, or 35% of the behaviors listed in the questionnaire. Nurses tended to perceive listening and discussing patients' feelings as relatively more important than patients did; and patients tended to perceive receiving physical care administered adequately and on time, and the nurse being friendly as relatively more important than the nurses did. These differences may simply reflect disagreement on the meaning of support as a semantic issue, or they may reflect differences in the priorities placed by nurses and patients on various nursing activities. If such a difference does exist, it may indicate that patients may not understand or agree to the importance of discussing their feelings with nurses to successful care outcomes as do nurses. Likewise, nurses may not understand or agree to the importance of having physical care administered adequately and on time and being friendly to patients to successful care outcomes as do patients.

The issue of whether or not nurses are currently perceived as placing too much or too little emphasis on each of these behaviors in their practice was not, of course, examined by this research. Although data analysis of this study is still preliminary and the practical implications of these findings are not entirely clear, they do provide a basis for tentatively concluding that patients and nurses place different priorities on certain supportive behaviors performed by nurses. There is also evidence that nurses tend to assign the same priority to the various supportive nursing activities regardless of specialty area, whereas patients tend to assign different priorities to some of the nursing supportive behaviors in the different specialty areas. Such differences in priorities suggest a potential for poor communication, and perhaps even discord between nurses and patients. Further research is indicated to determine whether or not the difference in priorities assigned to supportive behaviors found in this research constitutes a problem for effective care delivery and for nursing and patient education.

If the findings of this study are upheld with completed analysis of our data and further research is done to confirm these findings, these results may have an impact in nursing education and practice. The behaviors of the nurse could be taught and altered to conform more with the patients' perceived needs of being supported by the nurse. If patients perceive that they are being supported by the nurses, it is likely the patients' comfort and state of wellbeing will be enhanced.

References

1. Gardner: Supportive Nursing: A Critical Review of the Literature. Journal of Psychiatric Nursing and Mental Health Services, 17:6-10, October 1979.

Caring as the Focus of a Multidisciplinary Health Center for the Elderly

12

Joan Uhl, R.N., M.S.

A facility providing health services to elderly citizens residing in an urban area was primarily planned and implemented by four nursing faculty from the University of Utah College of Nursing. Boyle J, Uhl JE, and Day G (unpublished data, 1977), have described this nursing clinic, discussed its utilization by some elderly citizens, and evaluated the health maintenance aspects of the clinic. This health care facility was structured around the caring components and the open health care system model postulated by Leininger.[1-3] Since its inception four years ago (1975), this elderly health care service has expanded from a belief in the caring process held by four faculty members to a multidiscliplinary, open health care system that functions with a focus on caring processes as outlined by Leininger.[3]

The term *caring* was defined by Leininger[3] as that which "refers to the direct (or indirect) nurturant and skillful activities, processes, and decisions related to assisting people in such a manner that reflects behavioral attributes which are empathetic, supportive, compassionate, protective, succorant, educational, and otherwise dependent upon the needs, problems, values, and goals of the individual or group being assisted." These caring components will be discussed and the effectiveness of their application in an elderly health care center will be assessed later in this paper.

Open Health Care System Model

The open, client-centered health care system model proposed by Leininger[1] provides options for the elderly which allow the client to *select,* with assistance from the primary health care provider, the type of care most acceptable and accessible to himself (see Figure 12.1). This model used and discussed below for the elderly health center had many beneficial outcomes. The traditional health care system and roles of health professionals will be challenged in this paper as less preferable to Leininger's open health care model.

While the new open health care service was being operationalized, an independent study was conducted by a Salt Lake City Community Services Council to consider inclusion of health services for the

FIGURE 12.1

AN OPEN, CLIENT-CENTERED HEALTH CARE SYSTEM MODEL*

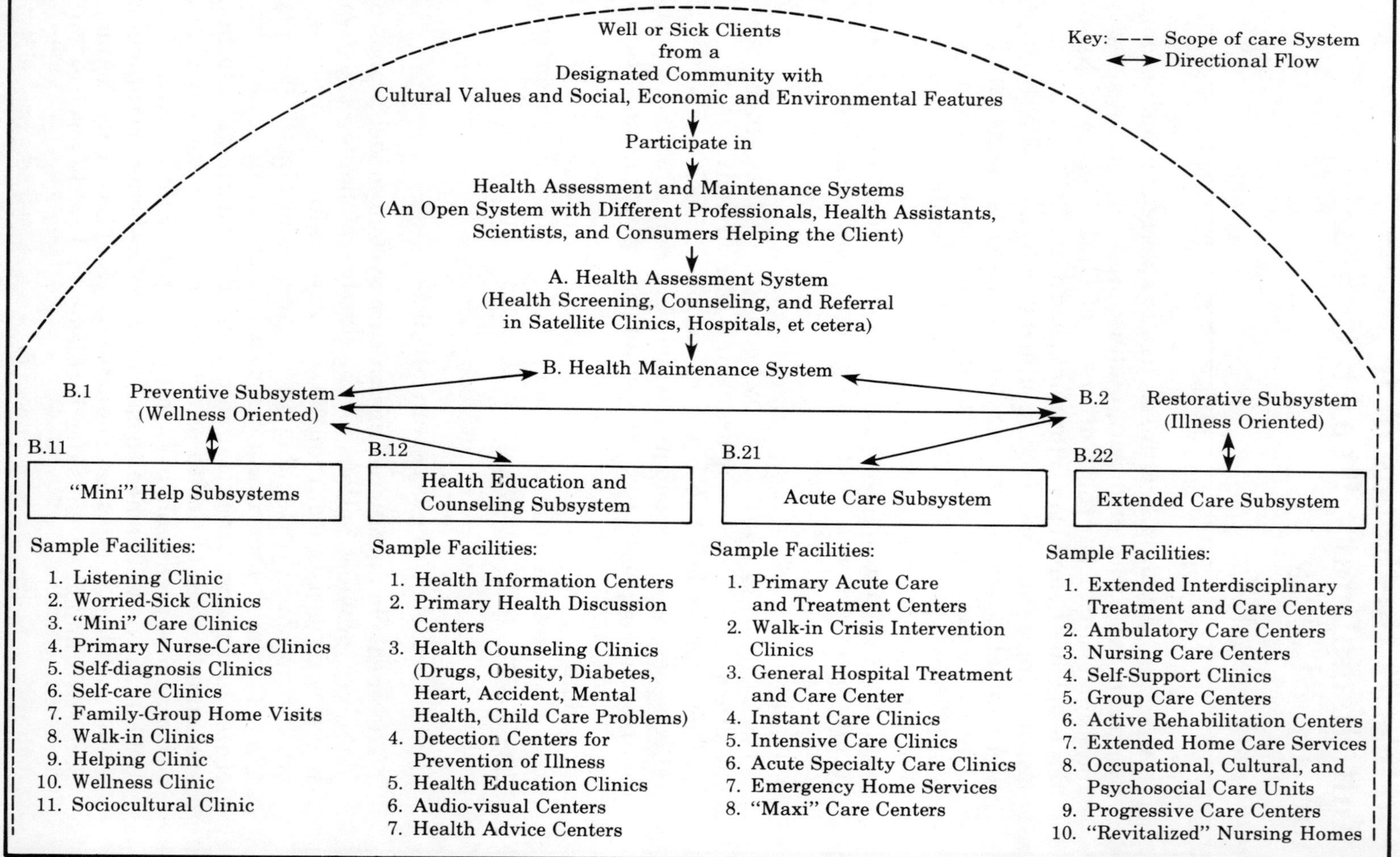

elderly residents of a soon-to-be-completed Housing and Urban Development high-rise apartment building. This study identified many unmet health needs of low-income elderly in central Salt Lake City and led to the submission of a grant proposal to implement research recommendations by establishing a permanent health care facility within a high-rise apartment building. This proposal was funded by the Intermountain Regional Medical Program, and was to be administered by the Rocky Mountain Gerontology Center at the University of Utah. The program administrator of the newly funded grant contacted the Dean of the College of Nursing to suggest some planning for collaboration with Rocky Mountain Gerontology Center and integration of the original nursing clinic and the proposed health center for elderly citizens. The caring components of the nursing clinic were identified and integrated in their entirety into the plans for an ideal health care facility for the elderly which would also provide an educational and research site for students and faculty from several university disciplines.

Initially, the Rocky Mountain Gerontology Center received funds to provide five areas of service to the elderly: 1) basic health screening services to the elderly within the high-risk as well as to others within Salt Lake County; 2) health education courses directed towards encouraging the elderly to become actively engaged in health care and nutrition; 3) basic first-aid training; 4) investigation of the possibilities of a pharmaceutical dispensary in the high-rise; and 5) assistance in obtaining transportation for the elderly to health care services. Many agencies and institutions have assisted in implementing some of these plans. The Salt Lake City and County Housing Authorities constructed the health center's facilities and leased them to the Rocky Mountain Gerontology Center for $1.00 per year. Costs for utilities and transportation for the elderly citizens to the center have been absorbed by the Salt Lake County Division for the Aging. Staffing for the entire project, with the exception of a full-time salaried project director and a part-time receptionist/secretary, has been provided by faculty and students of the various health and health-related disciplines of the universities involved.

The organizational structure of the multidisciplinary health center consists of:

1) *Project Administrator*—the principal investigator and grantee.
2) *Project Director*—a full-time salaried staff person.
3) *Advisory Committee*—the former Community Services Council planning committee members now constitute this committee. It is chaired by the project administrator and consists of ten members who represent the areas of nursing, medicine, social work, the Division of Aging, Salt Lake County Housing Authority, and consumers. Six of these ten members are senior citizens. The project director also serves on this committee. The function of this committee is to advise and discuss matters related to health care services for elderly clients living in the Salt Lake County area. The committee is routinely appraised by the project director of the functions and major changes in the health center and its services.

4) *Services and Programs Committee*—chaired by a committee member who also serves as an *ex-offico* member of the Advisory Committee. All members of this committee are faculty with the exception of the project director. Nursing students fulfilling their Nursing Management practicum requirements at this facility sit on this committee as *ex-offico* members.

The function of the Services and Programs Committee is to coordinate, plan, and direct the multidisciplinary services of the health center. At least one faculty member from each discipline currently utilizing the health center as a clinical/practicum faculty with either graduate or undergraduate students must serve on this committee. The Services and Programs Committee is the major planning and coordinating committee in the project. It provides direction and quality assurance for the entire health center. This committee has also been able to maintain the philosophy of the open health care system of health service to the elderly clients. This is attributable to the fact that this committee was chaired by the nurse-faculty member who helped to initiate the original nursing clinic on the above Leininger Model (Figure 12.1).

Student and faculty participation in the health center provides educational facilities for student placement and special opportunities for students to work with the elderly, insights into the benefits of collaborating with other health care services, and systematic study of phenomena related to health care for the elderly.

Health Center Location

The site selected for this center is a low-income high-rise apartment complex in central Salt lake City. It is centrally located near the greatest population of elderly citizens and readily accessible by public transportation. The center is also a major congregate meal site for senior citizens (Title VII Nutrition Program), and senior citizens from other congregate meal sites throughout the Salt Lake County are bused to the center for health care services. This transportation has been made available to elderly citizens who have heard about the health center as well as to the clients from the original high-rise site in which the first nursing clinic was established.

Client Population

Elderly citizens, aged 55 years or older, are the target population for this health center. The 350 residents of this apartment high-rise facility must meet Federal Housing and Urban Development guidelines for residency regarding level of income. It is interesting to note, however, that approximately two-thirds of the clients use the health center which is in the high-rise and surrounded by a community living area. Of those clients who have participated in the health center, over 65% have fixed annual incomes of $3,000 or less, and fewer than 15% have annual incomes of more than $5,000. Thus, the large majority of clients fall well below the poverty threshold as defined by Health, Education, and Welfare guidelines. To some, this might dictate the frequent use of the non-fee-for-service health center; however, the data show that the elderly citizens are satisfied with the services provided and are highly complementary of the humanistic and caring environment provided.

Demographics of Target Population

The 1970 Census counted 112,540 residents over the age of 60, and 77,500 over the age of 65 in the State of Utah. The latter group comprises 7.2% of the total population of the state, which is somewhat less than the 9.9% of the elderly in the U.S. population and is mainly attributable to the state's relatively high birth rate. Forty-five percent of the older population in Utah reside in Salt Lake County. Ethnic minorities comprise only 1.6% of the age 60 and over population in Salt Lake County. Of this 1.6% (n = 824) non-White older population, 30.7% are black and the remainder consist of Chicano, Native Americans, and Asian-Americans. The 1979 Census reported the total population breakdown of non-whites (n=8,826) in Utah shows 28% black, 18.3% Native American, 28.7% Japanese, 7.9% Chinese, 17% Filipino, and all other non-white populations 15.3%. Typically, older females outnumber males, with the disparity increasing with age.

The Multidisciplinary Health Care Team

Following growth and expansion of the original nursing clinic to provide health care for the elderly, one University of Utah nursing faculty member continued to plan and develop a multidisciplinary health care center for the elderly in collaboration with faculty and health care planners affiliated with the Rocky Mountain Gerontology Center. The conceptual design for care was to use the caring constructs found in the Transcultural Caring Model proposed by Leininger.[3] The College of Nursing and other disciplines from the University of Utah have had major representation and responsibility in the health center. Utah State University, Weber State College, and Brigham Young University faculty and students have participated to a lesser degree in this center. Currently, the multidisciplinary health center for the elderly provides services from the disciplines of nursing, family, and community medicine, pharmacy, social work, dietetics, dental hygiene, physical and occupational therapy, and leisure studies. Faculty and students provide services and use the health center for practicum placement for several courses.

Services offered by this multidisciplinary health care team center around the components of Leininger's health care system model as depicted above in Figure 12.1. The primary purpose of the health center is to assist the elderly to cope effectively with health problems and with the stresses of life, to facilitate health referrals, to provide health education, to promote health maintenance and illness prevention, and to provide general health screening services. All these services are provided by way of a humanistic caring process utilized across all disciplines.

Nursing Care for the Elderly

Nursing care is provided by faculty and undergraduate students in relation to the following courses: Community Health Nursing, Nursing Management, Psychosocial Nursing, and Nursing Research. Graduate students pursuing master and doctoral study in nursing also provide some services. The latter students come from the Family Nurse Clinician program, Gerontological Nurse Clinician program, and Psychosocial Nursing. The services and educational experiences include the following:

1) Interview and record health client histories with a culturological health assessment to identify how the clients are coping with the health programs and their pattern of health behaviors.
2) Provide physical examination (when necessary) to identify any gross health problems and assess the status of known health problems.
3) Identify alteration in human functioning.
4) Provide health promotion and illness prevention assessment and education.
5) Use of both inter- and intra-personal processes to clients through consultation and collaborative care models.
6) Collaborate with other disciplines in providing instrumental care related to diet and nutrition, exercise, elimination, medication, podiatry, and other health maintenance behaviors.
7) Screen clients for blood pressure, vision, hearing, and vital signs to detect problems that may require attention or referral to other health care professionals.
8) Make appropriate referrals to community agencies.
9) Evaluate emotional, social, economic, and educational needs.
10) Evaluate signs and symptoms that may be interfering with activities of daily living.
11) Provide therapeutic counseling, reassurance, and information related to stress, loneliness, mourning, and coping with health care problems.
12) Make referrals to a physician for medical care (after a clinic evaluation) and with the client's permission, or upon request.

Other Services

Dietetic

Services provided by faculty, undergraduate, and graduate students related to dietetics include the following:

1) Provide consultation related to therapeutic diets (eg, salt restricted, diabetic, low calorie) and caring needs.
2) Make nutritional assessments (eg, food intake, dietary evaluation, height, weight, and skinfold measurement).

Pharmacy

Services provided by faculty and doctoral students related to drugs and the pharmaceutical services include:

1) Record drug histories.
2) Counsel clients regarding medications, side-effects, and other aspects.
3) Encourage drug therapy compliance.
4) Provide health education programs related to medications and other toxic substances.

Physical and Occupational Therapy

Services provided by faculty, undergraduate, and graduate students in this area include:

1) Evaluate the range of client's motion.
2) Assess muscle strength of client.
3) Evaluate the performance and activities of client in daily living.
4) Evaluate sensory and perceptual status of the client.
5) Acquaint the client with adaptive equipment, methods to overcome architectural barriers, labor-saving devices, etc.

Social Work

Services provided by faculty and students related to social work include:

1) Identify community resources for the client.
2) Assist in client referral follow-up and compliance.
3) Participate in home visits with community health nursing students.
4) Participate in individual and group work with clients.

Leisure Studies

Services provided by faculty and students in areas of lesiure studies include:

1) Coordinate a variety of leisure time activities for clients.
2) Assist clients to program their own activities.
3) Counsel clients in use of their leisure time.
4) Assist clients with lifestyle development.

Dental Hygiene

Services provided by faculty and students in dental hygiene include:

1) Conduct oral soft tissue dental inspection.
2) Record oral hygiene indices.
3) Make referrals to other dentists or health care providers.
4) Conduct dental and oral health education programs.
5) Consult with other health care providers about client's dental needs.

Medicine

Services provided by faculty and students related to medicine are:

1) Performance of physical medication examinations.
2) Record taking of findings in POMR format.
3) Augment or assist nursing students to perform physical examinations.
4) Provide humanistic medical care.

Client Referral

This service is provided by all faculty and students participating in the health center for the elderly. This health care provides clients with assistance in the form of suggestions and options for follow-up care and referrals to any health or agency service desired by the client to the extent available. Extensive referral lists have been developed with the assistance of all disciplines in collaboration with community-based agencies staff and their resources.

Home Visits

Visits are made by nursing faculty, nursing, and social work students. Home visits have traditionally been made by community health nursing students to elderly citizens who reside in the high-rise and in the community who cannot come to the health center for any reason. Currently, social work students have been accompanying the nurse to assist as well as model the nursing care interventions.

Special Clinics

Other special clinical services for the elderly include:

1) Health education (a specific focus or topic per session).
2) Foot screening and referral.
3) Dental screening and referral.
4) Blood pressure screening and referral.
5) First aid instruction.
6) Immunizations.

In the 2½ year period this health center has been operating, over 2,200 clients have obtained health care.

The Caring Process and Research Potentials

According to Leininger,[3] caring "is the central unifying concept and essence of nursing theory and practice. Caring makes nursing unique and different in form, expression, and the content focus from other health care disciplines. . . ." The author's further reference to caring as the *primary* focus of nursing in contrast to medicine's unique and primary focus on curing processes, behaviors, and practices was made by Leininger. She challenges nurses to identify, define, classify, and refine ethnocaring constructs with the goal to gain and use cultural and sub-cultural values, health beliefs, caring practices, and other culture-specific characteristics. Leininger defined nursing as:

> ". . . the learned humanistic and scientific discipline which focuses upon caring behaviors, caring interactional processes, and caring skills of individuals, groups (culture and social), and community populations in order to assist people to attain and maintain a health status which is congruent with their cultural

values and with their psychosocial and physiological humanistic needs and life patterns."

In order to validate the caring constructs as described by Leininger in a nurse-centered, caring-oriented health facility for an elderly subculture, it is necessary to examine these definitions.

A subculture is defined as "a group that deviates in certain areas or features with respect to values, beliefs, and behavior from that of a dominant or parent culture with which they are perceived or known to be closely identified in daily life." Sullivan[4] utilized a framework suggested by Rose[5] in which the latter proposed the research theory of older people as a subculture as a unifying principle to study the aged. As a result of being considered old in our society, the elderly share certain situations and characteristics. Rose postulated that the emergence of a subculture of the aged has occurred because of the large number of people over 65, shared grievances, segregation by society into retirement communities and elderly high-rise apartments, and retirement encouraged at younger ages. The subsequent disengagement and disassociation from major social institutions leads to greater opportunity to interact and identify with each other in clubs and organizations, to congregate at meal sites for senior citizens, and to experience decreased contact with younger people. Rose concluded that the elderly subculture is characterized by values, beliefs, and behaviors distinctive to that group, namely, decreased emphasis on occupational prestige, increased emphasis on physical and mental health, increased interaction with each other and less with younger people, increased emphasis on leisure activities, and increased identification with members of their own age group.

Because clients utilizing the services of the health center for the elderly can be identified as a subculture, several of Leininger's nursing care hypotheses and propositions have possibilities for investigation:[3]

Identifiable differences in caring values and behaviors between and among cultures lead to differences in the nursing care expectations of care seekers.

Differences in caring values and norms of behavior exist between technologically dependent and non-technologically dependent societies and groups.

Professional people working in strange cultures with different values about nursing care or caring behaviors can create obvious cultural conflicts and problems unless they are willing to recognize and adapt to indigenous caring values and expectations.

The greater the dependence of nursing personnel upon technological caring tools and activities, the greater the interpersonal distance and the fewer the client's satisfactions.

The greater the differences between indigenous cultural caring values and modern professional nursing care values, the greater the signs of cultural conflict and stresses in caregiving and care receiving contexts.

Nursing care interventions which provide culture-specific caring practices will show greater signs of satisfaction from clients than will nonculturally oriented caring services.

Professional caring behaviors which are congruent with the social structure and the values of a particular culture or subculture will show greater client satisfaction and acceptance than those caring behaviors which show incogruencies with the values and social structure of a given culture.

Cultures and subcultures that have been traditionally dependent upon kinship groups for caring will expect more humanistic kinds of nursing care practices and less scientific-technological caregiving services.

The above Leininger hypotheses and propositions are being examined for investigation and inquiry into the aspects of caring behaviors of the nurse working with an elderly subculture. From such investigation, data may provide a basis for solving nursing problems and generating additional nursing theories to be tested. The descriptive data could be valuable as evidence of nursing as a discipline based on caring components. With empirically-based clinical and health care data and hypodeductive formulations about nursing care and caring behaviors, the body of knowledge in nursing could be firmly built and nursing care phenomena classified.

Accordingly, the authors designed a study related to caring behaviors of nurses who are working in health facilities for the elderly. These data will be compiled by a nurse researcher who is a participant-observer and who is using the Leininger ethnonursing model. Some of the care constructs to be studied (as identified by Leininger's research[3]), are the following: comfort and support measures, compassion, empathy, helping behaviors, coping behaviors, stress alleviation measures, touching, nurturance, succorance, surveillance, protective, restorative, and stimulative behaviors, health maintenance acts, health instruction, health consultation, and special ethnocare techniques.

To study the services and caring behaviors offered at the Health Center for the Elderly, some aspects of the caring model may be delineated. The Health Center is focused on the caring processes and other aspects of Leininger's model. Could one speculate that these caring constructs can be generalized and broadened to move beyond the specific nursing behaviors to affect the more universal health care program or to describe a health care system? Such speculation is not without basis for as we consider the Leininger Open Health Care Model, one can identify the caring constructs. This leads to further speculation that the discipline of nursing, if based on the caring components, may be represented as a model for health care systems. In the near future, the traditional health care system and roles of health professionals may be challenged by others. With the possible advent of national health insurance, the discrimination and inequality among health providers, (especially between physicians and nurses) may decrease. One may then further speculate about the long term effects of this change in the hierarchy and the possibility of the caring model and nursing care being adopted by consumers as their choice of health care system.

With the remarkable growth and acceptability of the Health Center for the Elderly in Salt Lake City in the past four years, this system of health care should be examined and evaluated by health care policy makers for future use. It has been suggested that because the health center for the elderly emphasizes health maintenance and illness prevention, and because nurses and other health personnel receive a reasonable fee for service, this type of facility would be cost-feasible and at the same time provide helpful, humanistic, competent, and nonfragmented health care.

Two other studies are being formulated by a nurse researcher and the project director of the Health Center for the Elderly which are related to subsets of the transcultural caring constructs. One is to examine and compare compliance behaviors of an elderly subculture in an open-system health center with those of a group of elderly citizens who utilize a traditional health care system. The research hypothesis is: There will be no significant difference in compliance behavior, related to referrals, between elderly citizens attending an open health care center and those seeking health care in a traditional health care facility.

The other study will examine student nurse caring behaviors and look for differences between those students who used a prescribed culturalogical assessment when interviewing elderly clients in an open-system health center, and those who did not use a prescribed culturalogical assessment. While these two studies are not too sophisticated nor complex in design or method, the author believes that involvement of student nurses in these types of studies will foster an interest in research and increase their awareness of caring behaviors. It will also help students to become less ethnocentric, and enhance interpersonal sensitivity, in addition to generating substantial knowledge about caring and the elderly.

References

1. Leininger M: An Open Health Care System Model. Nursing Outlook. 1972, 21, 1971-1975.
2. Leininger M: (ed.) Health Care Dimensions: Transcultural Health Care Issues and Conditions. Philadelphia, FA Davis, 1976.
3. Leininger M: Transcultural Nursing: Concepts, Theories, and Practices. New York, Wiley, 1978, pp 32, 33, 37, 38, 39, 40, 113.
4. Sullivan T: Some Values, Beliefs, and Practices of the Elderly in the United States: Implications for Health and Nursing Care. In Leininger M: (ed.), Transcultural Nursing Care of the Elderly. Proceedings from the Second National Transcultural Nursing Conference, University of Utah, Salt Lake City, Utah, 1977.
5. Rose AM: The Subculture of the Aging: A Framework for Research in Social Gerontology. In Rose, AM Peterson WA: (eds.): Older People and Their Social World. Philadelphia, FA Davis, 1965.

Part III — 1980

Characteristics and Classification of Caring Phenomena

Third National Caring Conference

March 18, 19, 1980
University of Utah
Salt Lake City, Utah

Caring From a Human Science Perspective

13

*Rosemarie Rizzo Parse, R.N., Ph.D.**

This paper will address the concept of caring from a human science perspective. It will examine caring as a function of healing in light of culturally grounded value systems. Caring will be discussed relative to its essential elements: risking, being-with, and moment of joy. The phenomenological research method will be discussed as well as implications for curriculum to study care in families.

Tenets of the Human Science Nursing

In order to understand caring from a human science perspective, it is important to explore briefly the basic tenets of human science nursing theory. The author's human science nursing is an emerging theory which posits beliefs about man, living, and health.[1,2] These beliefs are made explicit through the language peculiar to the theory. For the purpose of achieving common understanding, the following terms are defined and briefly discussed.

Living unity—refers to man's† wholeness. This means that man is more than and different from the sum of his parts. The critical essence of wholeness is in the meaning of *more than,* which illuminates man's relationship with the environment. Man's wholeness cannot be known through a study of his parts. Man-environment cocreates patterns of expression through which man is recognized.

Negentropy—refers to the concept of negative entropy, which posits growth as multidimensional and moving toward increasingly complex and heterogeneous dimensions. Health is man's negentropic unfolding.

Freedom-in-situation—refers to man always being free in a situation. In and through his choices, man gives meaning to his world. He bears responsibility for choices and lives the consequences of his decisions. The options from which man chooses are always contextual in nature in that they arise from miltidimensional experiences.

**This is a synopsis of the author's presentation, given at the Third National Caring Conference.*

†*No distinction is made with respect to gender in this paper.*

Intersubjectivity—refers to an encounter between two human subjects. Martin Buber defines the sphere of the between where two human subjects encounter each other in a dynamic process of becoming.[3] This encounter is an open, honest, authentic presence where each is confirmed and affirmed by the other.

Coexistence—refers to man's existence being only through coexistence. Man's humanness is confirmed only in relation with other human beings.

Coconstitution—refers to the coauthoring of relationships in which participants choose a way of being in a situation with each other. This way of being cocreates the emerging relationship as it continuously unfolds in the betweeness of the participants.

The central phenomenon of human science nursing is man-living-health. Nursing concerns itself with the client's lived experience of health as reflected in patterns of expression. Assumptions about man and health are specified. Health is conceptualized as an open process of being-becoming experienced by the client. Man and environment move mutually and simultaneously in cocreating changing patterns of the health situation. Health as man's pattern of expressing value priorities in a situation proposes that man's values are incarnated in his choices. Man continuously reaches out, choosing health possibilities, and in the choosing moves toward the possible. The movement is multidimensional and toward greater complexity and heterogeneity.

Human science nursing posits man as open, synergistic, and free-in-situation, coconstituting the world in coexistence with others.[2,5] That man experiences coexistence while coconstituting rhythmical patterning with the environment means that man and environment move together mutually and simultaneously in the inevitable "ebb and flow of the dance of life." Man as a thinking, feeling, open being has the freedom to choose in situations and to bear responsibility for his decisions. Man cannot not choose though choices are made without knowing either the full range of options or the full range of consequence. Man creates patterns of expression in a coconstituted way of being with others, and it is through these patterns of expression that he is known. Man's patterns of expression are unique, ever changing, yet recognizable. Man lives in continuing movement beyond the actual toward the possible. This movement is unidirectional and multidimensional toward greater complexity.

Definition of Caring

With this as background, a definition of caring could be stated as follows: ***caring** is risking being with someone towards a moment of joy.* The essences that unfold from this synthesis are *risking, being with,* and *moment of joy.*

***Risking** is defined as being exposed to possible injury.* In relationships, risking is choosing originality in the way of being with the other in the mutual struggle toward growth. For the nurse, risking is coconstituting with a client in an open, authentic relationship through which both can grow. It is choosing to value the client as subject though the client's values are not necessarily those of the nurse. Inherent in the meaning of this essence is the subject-to-subject way of being with the client in which the nurse chooses to reach out to the client's call even though the reaching exposes the nurse to change and possibly, to hurt and rejection. The risking for the nurse and for the client lies in growing toward the possible, as well as in the possibility for rejection.

Being with *is encountering or reflectively attending to the other.* For the nurse, it is choosing to enounter the client in an open, authentic engagement. It is a way of reaching out to understand the client's experience. The nurse is authentically present in her/his wholeness to the wholeness of the client. The nurse as subject relates to the client as subject. The nurse bears a responsibility for choosing to participate with clients in the context of a health-related situation. Each experience of participation is a source of self revelation toward growth for both nurse and client.

Moment of joy *is the complementary rhythm of suffering-joying all at once.* The nurse, in risking to be with the client in a health-related situation for growth, shares in the client's suffering-joying. As the realization of the meaning of risking to be with another surfaces, suffering-joying emerges toward moment of joy. The nurse, bearing witness to the client's suffering-joying, coconstitutes moving toward the possible with the client. The nurse synchronizes energies with the client, through suffering-joying, to transcend toward greater complexity. The experience of suffering-joying is a simultaneous phenomenon lived as a part of the caring process.

As these essences—*risking, being with,* and *moment of joy*—are lived, healing unfolds in the intersubjective process of caring. Healing, choreographed by the nurse-client interrelationship, is the continuity of change that unfolds in the emergence and transformation toward a chosen direction. The chosen direction is articulated by the client as the nurse participates with the client in the unfolding of his desired patterns of health. These patterns of health are reflected in the relationship that exists between the client's past, present, and future. This connectedness unfolds in each movement and can be understood only by understanding the client as more than and different from the sum of his parts. It is in his wholeness and uniqueness that the client experiences healing through caring.

The etymology of the word *healing* refers to making whole or sound. Healing, as a process of little birthings and dyings, in coexistence with the nurse, a caring presence, cocreates transforming and transcending toward the possible. In this way healing emerges from caring.

Research Method: Phenomenology

The primary research method to uncover modes of caring in families from a human science perspective is the phenomenological method. ***Phenomenology*** *is a method of inquiry which focuses on the unfolding of a phenomenon as it is lived.* It is hypothesis generating. Through a rigorous dwelling with a phenomenon, the structure of a lived experience is uncovered.

To compare and contrast different modes of caring, it is suggested that persons from various cultural groups such as Italian, Polish, Jewish, and Irish, be invited to share situations in which they experienced *being cared for.* The phenomenological method would allow for the unfolding of a structure with each cultural group. The structures of being cared for from the various cultural groups could then be compared for similarities and differences. Hypotheses could be generated and further research studies designed and implemented.

Caregivers from the various cultural groups mentioned above might be invited to share situations in which they experienced caring for another. A similar comparison could be made, thereby unfolding the lived experience of caring for another. Through phenomenological method, the essence of caring as a lived experience in families in a multicultural society could be unfolded. This research would guide practice and enhance theory development in nursing.

Curricula at both graduate and undergraduate levels could be designed with a deliberate focus on the concept of caring. The emphasis would begin in the philosophy and be present thematically throughout the structure of the curricula. The concept of caring would be reflected in the goals, in the themes and level indicators, as well as with specific cultural content of courses.

References

1. Parse RR: Nursing Fundamentals. New York, Medical Examination Publishing Company, 1974.
2. Parse RR: Rights of Medical Patients. In Fischer C (ed): Client Participation in Human Services. New Brunswick, NJ, Transaction Books, 1978.
3. Buber M: I and Thou. New York, Charles Scribner's Sons, 1970.
4. Rogers M: An Introduction to the Theoretical Basis of Nursing. Philadelphia, FA Davis, 1970.

Some Philosophical, Historical, and Taxonomic Aspects of Nursing and Caring in American Culture

14

Madeleine Leininger, R.N., Ph.D., Lh.D., F.A.A.N.

As the nursing profession increasingly shows signs of maturity in academic scholarship, research, and teaching, and then translates this knowledge into professional practice, its members will realize the importance of domains of knowledge to explain and support the discipline of nursing. During the past two decades my writings, research, and conference leadership on caring has opened many new vistas for nurse researchers and theoreticians.[1-7] Since such pioneering work, more nurse researchers are pursuing diverse lines of inquiry regarding aspects of care behaviors, processes, and patterns of behavior with concommitant nursing care practices. This is an encouraging and exciting development, and one which is long overdue in nursing: to establish nursing as a full-fledged academic discipline and profession by emphasizing its central focus and essence.

There is, however, a continued need for rigorous and systematic study of care and caring by nurses, to discover the multifaceted aspects of care for quality nursing practices. It is also needed for other academic and professional disciplines to integrate the care construct into their research, teaching, and helping services as a critical and essential dimension of human relatedness and expression. It is my contention that all human beings need care for self-actualization, growth, and survival. The nursing profession should give leadership to explicate the concept of care as central to human living, maintenance of wellness, restoration of health, and many other human relatedness functions.

In this paper, I will provide some arguments and a rationale for ***caring*** *as the central, unique and unifying focus of nursing,* by looking at some logical and inferred deductions from our cultural history, philosophy, and the direction of nursing interests. A historical overview of some comparative linguistic useages of the term *care* will be presented. A structural taxonomic model to order and classify caring data, and to generate theories about caring will be presented, along with a suggested taxonomy on care.

Caring: A Reaffirmation and New Focus for Nursing

For more than two decades, I have emphasized that care is the essence and central focus of nursing. My cultural care investigation of 30 cultures helps to reaffirm the potential and to make care the distinctive feature of nursing. The full study of care offers great promise to make nursing a justified and respected discipline and profession. I have urged other nurses to pursue investigations on multiple aspects of care so that we can fully know the nature, scope, and functions of care relative to nursing. In another publication, I wrote:[5]

> One of the most essential, promising and important areas of study in nursing is the concept of caring. And yet, it has been one of the most neglected areas for systematic research. Although nurses are the professional group who repeatedly use the expressions *nursing care, care,* and *caring* in everyday parlance, the linguistic, semantic, and professional useages of these terms are limitedly understood and studied.

As a consequence of promoting the study of care, I find more nurses and nurse researchers are now focusing on the phenomenon of care or caring. Nursing students in graduate programs and some nursing faculty are beginning to realize the potentials in the study of the epistemological, linguistic, and cultural usages of care. I would predict that soon, medicine and other health disciplines will also pursue this line of inquiry. But most importantly, nurses need to focus on care. I believe nurses are coming of age to know the special characteristics and boundaries of the discipline of nursing through the care construct. Moreover, some faculty in schools of nursing are using caring as a major teaching construct and focus in teaching and research. This is encouraging to see nursing curricula changed from a medical model in the past, to a nursing care focus today. I see an awakening, a challenge, and a major new thrust in nursing as nurses study care and caring as a generic construct related to nursing care practices. Indeed, caring phenomenon has been obscure in nursing for many decades, and yet it is repeatedly used as an action modality and a linguistic explanation (or justification) by many nurses. Likewise, nursing faculty talk about *care* and *nursing care* in the classroom, but without explicating the characteristics and denotive aspects of care.

Not having explicated and tested concepts about caring, nurses have relied on medical curing, diagnostic, and treatment modes. Moreover, many nurse researchers tend to study medical phenomena and pathological symptoms, and give less attention to caring behaviors and processes. In the last five years, master and doctoral nursing students have begun to value and pursue research studies on caring and its relationship to nursing behaviors. For example, master and doctoral students at the University of Utah have been studying caring phenomenon—and especially transcultural nursing—for the past five years. Students are conducting indepth studies on care to build a body of knowledge in nursing that reflects empirical, symbolic, and ideal aspects of nursing. Most encouraging has been the work of transcultural nursing students who are focusing on comparative caring phenomenon. For example, Boyle's study on caring values and behaviors of the Chinese and Guatemalan nurses is a substantive and valuable piece of research.[8] Ray's work on institutional care in a hospital system has recorded some interesting facts about caring.[9] Other transcultural nursing students are studying particular care concepts such as support, nurturance, tenderness, touch, and comfort. The psychosocial, cultural, and physical aspects of these constructs, as seen from a holistic and ethnographic perspective, provides fresh insights about caring and health care practices cross-culturally. At the seven National Transcultural Nursing Conferences and the National Caring Conferences, the focus has been largely on caring, which has provided seminal ideas about comparative caring modes.[3,10,14] Thus, a new teaching, practice, and research ethos on the scientific and humanistic dimensions of caring is gradually emerging in nursing. It may well be that this interest in caring will grow in our schools of nursing, and in nursing practice. I am hopeful that by 1990 we will have substantive caring content with which to teach and guide nursing practice.

Philosophical and Historical Arguments for Caring

In answer to the question: "Why should nurses select caring as the dominant focus of nursing," I have found at least three substantive arguments. First, I believe historically, humans have needed caring throughout their life span, not only for their development and survival, but to meet life stresses and to develop as human beings. Caring attitudes and activities tend to stimulate human qualities in communication and relationship with other humans. Through a caring attitude, people are willing to share, be involved with, and concerned about others. Interestingly, anthropologists had not studied caring phenomenon until nurse-anthropologists entered the field. Now nurse-anthropologists are studying the evolutionary, functional, and historical aspects of caring, its importance to human survival and human development, and its ability to maintain wellness and to restore health.[5,15,16]

A second argument for caring is that with the rise of industrialism and technology, individuals appear to be getting less interpersonally and more materialistically oriented than ever before. Where is the increase in technological usage leading human beings in survival and living modes? From many indications, technological forms and modes of living will increase and not decrease. Since the danger of machine-like behavior in maintaining wellness and dealing with sickness seems imminent, all caregivers need to reflect upon the short and long range consequences of overuse and abuse of technologies in human health status. If humans live only for the present and neglect their race as well as their environment in the future, they are taking a short-sighted and noncaring attitude for the continuance of the species.

A third argument for nurses and others to support caring is that it denotes attitudes and activities of human service. To remove care from the title of health care services is like taking quality from the essence of any product or service. Caring for others by showing a genuine interest in, or an involvement with another person's life or condition remains essential to human services, and especially for health care. Nothing can quite replace human caring reflected in the capacity of an individual engaging in the aid of another individual, family, or community group in time of need, stress, or illness. What would nursing services be like if care were excluded from the service? The *nursing care* phrase has been used as a linguistic slogan for many decades. What does caring mean to nurses, physicians, and other health professionals? What research documents the characteristics and unique features of nursing care from other types of care? Frequently nurses say care is a personalized and benevolent act toward human beings in need of help. Does this idea give nursing its desired, distinctive, and unique feature? Is care always personalized and direct?

Nursing with caring attitudes and actions reflected in concern, helpfulness, compassion, protection, and other attributes assists individuals to recover from illness, stress, and life threats. Care, derived from *cura,* denotes concern for, commitment (or devotedness) to another, and attending to others.[12] A caring relationship, concern, and attitude have been important in the help of others. There is a sense of commitment and dedication in helping others through caring. Without caring a cold, indifferent, and mechanistic attitude exists toward people. Caring should be the hallmark or desired quality of nursing service. Care should be explicitly manifest to clients so that they are aware of caring services by nurses. If care remains obscure and assumed, then one can predict that the quality of human health and nursing services will be questionable, unsatisfactory, or non-therapeutic. Thus the rationale for the importance of care as a therapeutic and epistemological basis in nursing seems crucial, along with research to validate the above theoretical premises. In industrial language, the quality of the nursing "product" must show that care is included to assure that the product will be recognized by the public, and that it is respected, and economic. At this point in nursing, care is not a known and tested product.

Ten Premises and Questions to Guide Caring and Nursing Care Research

The following major premises and key questions may help to guide nurses to critically study caring as part of nursing services, research, and teaching:

1) Care and culture are closely linked.
2) Human caring is essential to human expression, relatedness to others, and for health needs and survivial.
3) The essential attributes, expressions, meanings, and processes of care can be identified, transmitted, and used in present-day nursing, teaching, and practice.

4) Professional nursing care must visibly and cognitively reflect direct and indirect *personalized caring* for therapeutic care to occur.
5) Caring is the generic component of all nursing service, and without therapeutic caring attitudes, expressions, and activities, nursing services are incomplete, mechanistic, inadequate, and questionable.
6) Human caring is culturally derived and therefore, nurses will need knowledge of the cultural values, beliefs, and practices of clients, families, and community groups to know and use caring therapeutically.
7) Human caring has nonverbal forms of expression which are extremely important to the care of people—perhaps more important than verbal expressions.
8) There is an art and science of caring which has both humanistic and scientific dimensions.
9) The relationship between caregivers and care recipients is limitedly known, and yet this relationship appears to be the heart of therapeutic help to clients.
10) Cross-cultural universal and non-universal caring values and practices are fairly obscure, and yet they remain the basis for all future nursing practices, education, and research modes.

Ten important research questions to be studied in nursing are as follows:

1) What was the cultural historical basis for generic human caring and nursing care, and how has caring changed through human evolution?
2) How critical is caring for human survival, development, and wellbeing through time and in different places in the world?
3) What are the cross-cultural universal and non-universal features of human caring?
4) What are the linguistic, social, and professional usages of care/caring in Western and non-Western cultures?
5) How is caring linked with social structure (eg, political, economic, kinship, religion)?
6) What theories of caring would explain professional and nonprofessional nursing care practices?
7) What essential characteristics denote caring and nursing care in different cultures?
8) What are the essential differences between caring and curing processes?
9) What cross-culture taxonomy could be used to order and study care phenomenon?
10) Why has the care/caring phenomenon been limitedly investigated in nursing in the past?

Taxonomy Model to Study Types of Care Phenomenon

As the body of nursing knowledge about care and caring, based upon knowledge of today and the anticipation of the future begins to grow, Figure 14.1 has been developed to help nurses conceptualize, order, and study types of caring phenomenon. With a taxonomy on care/caring, several purposes or benefits become apparent: 1) it helps to readily identify the broadest aspects of

FIGURE 14.1

LEININGER'S CONCEPTUAL AND THEORY-GENERATING MODEL TO STUDY TRANSCULTURAL AND ETHNOCARING CONSTRUCTS*

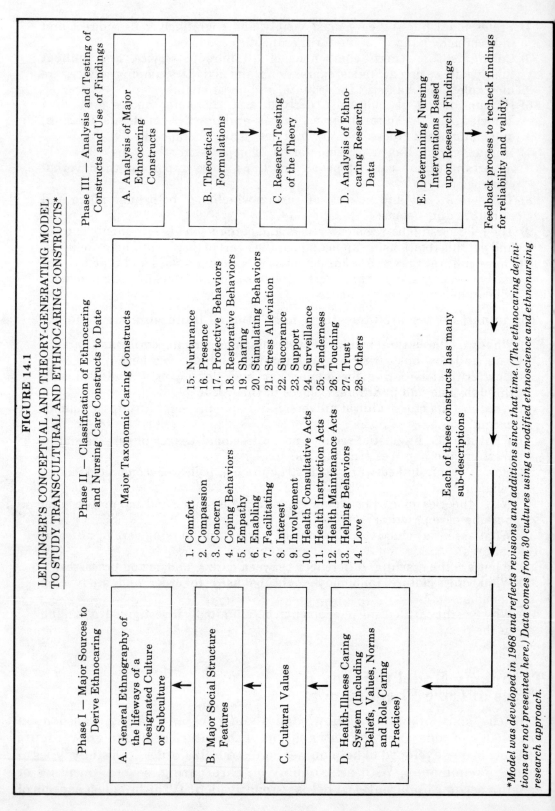

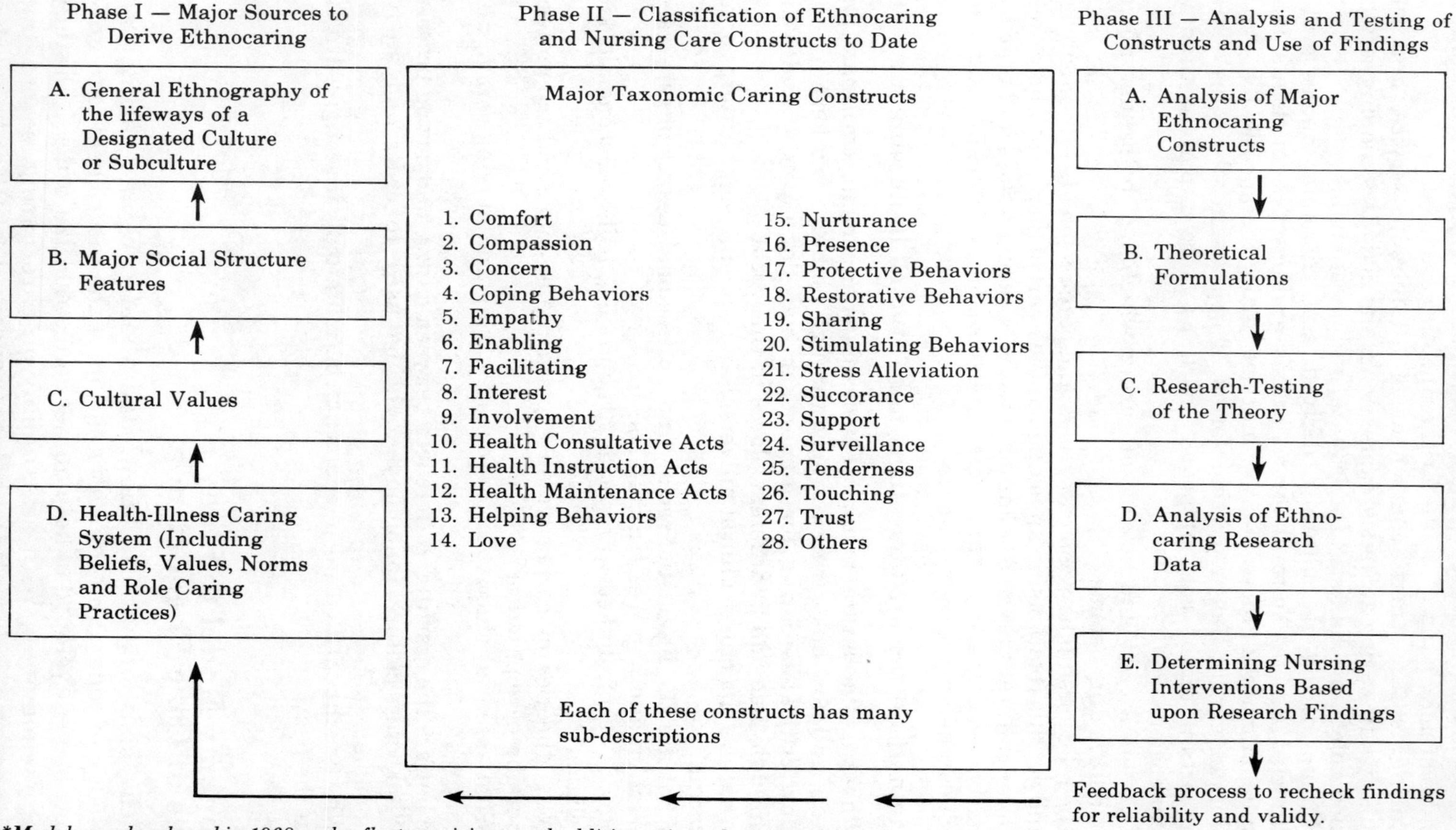

Model was developed in 1968 and reflects revisions and additions since that time. (The ethnocaring definitions are not presented here.) Data comes from 30 cultures using a modified ethnoscience and ethnonursing research approach.

the construct of care/caring; 2) it provides an orderly mode to classify and learn the different types of a phenomenon in relation to caring phenomenon; 3) it stimulates theorists and researchers to explore diverse variables about care (areas unexplored or open for study become apparent with a taxonomy); and 4) it provides a guide to generate nursing theories and research studies. In general, a taxonomy of any subject—and in this case with caring—has these general features: 1) it is an orderly way to arrange and study data at an early, evolving, or final stage of a matter; 2) it provides a conceptual structure to determine what is included or excluded on the subject; 3) it provides a ranking of large and small units of a phenomenon with subcategories according to knowledge about each domain; and 4) it reflects a dynamic or change structure to accommodate new knowledge about the phenomenon under study.[13]

Linguistic and Historical Usage of Care in the USA

In the United States, the concept of care and caring is being used more frequently in the literature by different health providers and by business organizations. But in many usages, the term is still vague. The function and meaning of slogans about caring is everyone's guess. The mystical and mythical aspects of care are quite evident in verbal discourses about nursing and health services. "Good caring", "true caring", and therapeutic care" are perceived quite differently by many professionals and non-professionals. In my interviews and discussions with professional nurses, they continue to use the term *care* when talking about *nursing care;* however, the meaning, and function of care is vague, and varies considerably among nurses. Furthermore, several older nurses said that they believe there are signs of a less caring attitude today than in the past. They find more technical care being given and less personalized care than in earlier days. These nurses add that since my writings have appeared in nursing literature and other places, they find there is a new or renewed interest in care and its relationship to nursing. In general, many nurses believe that a focus on caring is much needed today to improve personalized nursing care and to improve health care services.

Many conflicts exist in today's hospitals with well-intended nurses who value direct caring activities and attitudes, yet are pressed to monitor clients' physical conditions using electronic machines, provide various communications to physicians and others, do paper work, and attend meetings. The reason for the nursing shortage is unclear, but we know many nurses are dissatisfied with the conditions, salaries, and diverse role expectations. Furthermore, my cross-cultural findings reveal that nurses are largely taking care of physical stress alleviation and technological care in the United States. When large numbers of clients come to the hospital, a shortage of nursing staff occurs and only the most basic services are performed for the clients.

We need more nurse-administrators in top decision-making and policy roles who are committed to help nurses *give care.* They should not have to give physician care or perform housekeeping tasks. Nurses who know and value caring will have to emphasize caring as nursing. Nursing administrators need to organize and plan strategies to help nurses give care rather than partial technological, physical, or physican medical treatments. Where is therapeutic nurse care manifest and how does one assess and provide quality care? Nurses should also watch that they are not victims of technocracy and slaves to medical diagnostic and treatment regimens. The exploitation of women is well-known in the health fields, where it seems to be traditional to not value women in caregiving roles. It appears time to stem the current tide of technological and physical client services and to start to incorporate the broad psychosocial, cultural, and other aspects of caring practices into routine patient services. It is also my thesis that much of nursing dissatisfaction and burnout today is directly related to nurses not being able to give care in the fullest way desired and to receive positive rewards or recognition for their caring activities and efforts.

Linguistic Usages of Caring by Nurses and Physicians

In a cursory review of literature, the linguistic usages of the term *care* by nurses, physicians, and the public since the days of Nightingale were found, and are presented in Figure 14.2. I relied on samplings from the major professional journals in nursing and medicine, ie, *American Journal of Nursing, Nursing Outlook, American Journal of Medicine,* and *Journal of Public Health.* There were several findings that can be summarized:

1) Since the Nightingale days (post-1865), the nursing profession has consistently used the term *care* in their literature. The term is usually not defined, but linked as a suffix to nursing. There is usually no differential between *nursing* and *caring,* and these terms are often interchangeable.
2) From Figure 14.2, it can be seen that the nursing profession has the largest number of referent modifiers to *care* (eg, private care, hospital care, team care, primary care). Thus, by sheer linguistic usage, nurses have consistently used *care* for more than a century.
3) Physicians have used the term *care* more during the past three decades, and after nurses used it. The term *care* is being used with *medical care,* but without linguistic and semantic clarification.
4) The literature suggests that the terms *diagnosis, medical symptoms, pathologies,* and *medical curing* are used far more often by physicians than *care* or *caring.*
5) Since 1970, there have been more varient linguistic care referents used by nurses, and since that time, the study of caring has begun.
6) The public's use of the term *care* has not been explicit in literature. The public's linguistic and historical usage of care is used in such ways as: *being under my doctor's care, physician care, medical care* and *sick care.* The public does not use *nursing care* or *caring* in this literature.

Other fascinating professional and social usages related to care are being analyzed by the author.

FIGURE 14.2

RECURRENT LINGUISTIC USAGE OF *CARE* BY U.S. NURSING AND MEDICAL PROFESSIONS SINCE 1860*†

PERIOD	NURSING PROFESSION	MEDICAL PROFESSION	PUBLIC USAGE
1865-1930	Environmental (Care) Nursing Care Public Health Care	Limited use of care. More emphasis on diagnosis pathology, treatments, and curing terms.	Medicine (Services)*** Institutions
1930-50	*** Bedside Care Patient Care Custodial Care Individual Care Private Duty Care Medical and Nursing Care	*** Institutional Care Medical Care Hospital Care Individual Care Custodial Care	*** Institutional (Services)** Doctor (Help)** Hospital (Care) Medical Care
1950-60	*** Comprehensive Care Total Care Physical Care Hospital Care	*** Bedside Care Medical Care Medical Services Preventive Health Care	*** Private Care "Doctor" (Care) Home Care Hospital Care
1960-70	*** Interdisciplinary Care Community Mental Health Care Community Nursing Care Primex & Primary Care Distributive-Episodic Care	*** Community Medical Care Hospital Team Care Interdisciplinary Care Technical Care Medex Medicare & Medicaid Care	*** Home Nursing (Care Scientific Medical Care Medical Treatments Medicare Insurance Care
1970-80	*** Scientific-Technical Care Self-Care Humanistic Care Quality Care Health Maintenance Care Health Care Preventive Nursing Care Transcultural Nursing Care Ethical Care Holistic or Wholistic Care	*** Preventive Medical Care Primary Care Ethical-Moral (Care) Quality Care Holistic Care	*** Ethical (Care) Care to Poor Human Care

Code: Arrow (▼) indicates historical sequencing in care use.
**Detailed analysis of literature in process. This reflects preliminary survey.*
***Infers attributes of care in context fo discussion.*
****Includes above section in adition to the terms below.*
†Copyrighted by Madeleine Leininger, 1981.

To conclude this section, Figure 14.3 is offered as a suggested taxonomy on care to help nurses order and classify types of caring or care phenomenon. As a suggested framework, it can be used as a guide to classify future knowledge through research studies.

FIGURE 14.3

LEININGER'S SUGGESTED TAXONOMY OF CARE/CARING*†

Purposes of Taxonomy: 1) To provide an orderly classification to evolving forms and expressions of care and caring; 2) To build a body of caring knowledge; and 3) To generate theories and research on caring.

I. *Universal Care Types and Attributes*
   A. Prehistorical human care
   B. Historical human care

II. Cultural Specific Care Types and Attributes
   A. Western Cultures
   B. Non-Western Cultures

II. *Transcultural Emic-Etic Care Relationships***
   A. Emic and Etic Western Care Types
      1. Folk Care Types
      2. Professional Care Types
   B. Emic and Etic Non-Western Care Types
      1. Folk Care Types
      2. Professional Care Types
   C. Other features — Western and Non-Western Types

IV. *Health Professional and Non-Professional Care Attributes*
   A. Health Professional Care Types
      1. Nursing Care Provider Types
      2. Non-Nursing Care Provider Types
   B. Non-Professional Health Care Providers
      1. Special Types
      2. Universal Types

V. *Social Structure and Individual Group Care Types and Relationships*
   A. Social Structure Types
      1. Economic Care
      2. Political and Legal Care
      3. Kinship Care
      4. Technological Care
      5. Cultural Group Values
   B. Individual and Group Care
      1. Individual Care
      2. Group Care
   C. Other Forms of Care
      1. Institutional Care
      2. Non-institutional Care
      3. Humanistic Care Types
      4. Scientific Care Types

**Developed in 1967 with added additions and modifications.*
***Emic — refers to the local or native point of view about a phenomenon under study.*
Etic — refers generally to universal aspects of a phenemenon under study.
†Copyrighted by Madeleine Leininger, 1981.

VI. *Transcultural Nursing Care by Specific Cultures*
- A. North American
- B. South American
- C. African
- D. Oceania
- E. Southeast Asia
- F. Middle East
- G. Caribbean
- H. Other

VII. *Interdisciplinary Care Types*
- A. Nursing Care Types
- B. Medical Care Types
- C. Social Work Care Types
- D. Others

VIII. *Other Types of Care and Relation to Cure Types*

References

1. Leininger M: The Essence of Nursing: Caring. Read at the American Nurses Convention, New Jersey, 1967.
2. Leininger M: The Changing Role of the Nurse. Read at the Washington State Medical Association Annual Meeting, Seattle, Washington, September 19, 1972.
3. Leininger M: Humanistic Care: An Alive, Dormant or Lost Art? Read at the Seventh Annual Maryam Smith Memorial Lecture, University of Utah, Salt Lake City, Utah, May 25, 1973.
4. Leininger M: Transcultural Nursing: Concepts, Theories, and Practices. New York, John Wiley & Sons, 1978.
5. Leininger M: The Phenomenon of Caring. American Nurses' Foundation (Nursing Research Report), Vol 12, No 1, February, 1977.
6. Leininger M: The Phenomenon of Caring: Research Questions and Theoretical Considerations. Read at the First National Caring Conference, University of Utah, Salt Lake City, Utah, April 1978.
7. Leininger M: Caring: The Central Essence and Nature of Professional Nursing. Read at the 1978 Centennial Symposium, Duquesne University School of Nursing, Pittsburgh, Pennsylvania, October 28, 1978.
8. Boyle J: Nursing Care in the People's Republic of China. Presented at University of Utah, Salt Lake City, Utah, 1979.
9. Ray M: Study of Institutional Caring Behaviors. Study in progress for Doctoral Dissertation Requirements, University of Utah, College of Nursing, Salt Lake City, Utah, 1979-80.
10. Leininger M: Caring: The Essence and Focus of Nursing. Proceedings of the Three National Caring Conferences, Salt Lake City, Utah, 1980.
11. Leininger M: Futurology of Nursing: Goals and Challenges for Tomorrow. In Chaska N (ed):Views Through the Mist: The Nursing Profession. New York: McGraw-Hill Book Co, 1978.
12. Partridge E: Origins: A Short Etymological Dictionary of Modern English. New York: MacMillan Co, 1958, p 135.
13. Leininger M: Introduction to Taxonomic Principles of Caring. Read at the Third National Conference, Salt Lake City, Utah, March 19, 1980.
14. Leininger M: Proceedings of the National Transcultural Nursing Conferences. New York, Masson International Publishing Company, 1979.
15. Watson J: Nursing: The Philosophy and Science of Caring. Boston, Little, Brown & Co, 1979.
16. Amaodt AM: The Care Component in a Health and Healing System. In Bauwens E (ed): The Anthropology of Health. St. Louis, CV Mosby Co, 1978.

Reflections on the Biopolitics of Human Nature and Altruism*

15

P. Morley, Ph.D.

Recent developments in social biology have raised a number of controversial issues concerning the nature of mankind.† The biological rule of genetic determinism, as exemplified in the work of Wilson[1] and Dawkins[2] has reintroduced the problem of human nature couched in scientific terms, and seemingly devoid of metaphysical uncertainly. The nature-nurture debate is critically examined by the sociobiologists with a view to demonstrating that such human values as altrusim, mortality, religion, and love are but the survival strategies of our "selfish genes", which have travelled an evolutionary path preceding our individual human existence. In this paper I examine the fundamental issues of the new biology in an attempt to elucidate the nature of human nature and its implications for caring.[3] In essence, my thesis is that this biologist perspective emerges as a powerful new force in social theory, a force which gives impetus to deterministic notions of human potential, and which may be seen as the theoretical *chic* of contemporary Social Darwinism. The philosophy of caring (and its praxis) may now be debated within the scientific arena. Is this science or scientism? This paper reflects on our genetic predisposition to care or not to care.

On Human Nature

The nature of man is a central problem for the development of a science of man. The question of whether man is inherently good or evil, or simply neutral, is fundamental to both the shape and direction of the human sciences, for these must be influenced "by the image of man at its center."[4] If, for example, we assert that man is good, then *ab initio* we have one kind of science. Should we, on the other hand, decide that man is inherently evil, then we have a different type of science—one that is diametrically opposed to the first. Our points of departure clearly shape our hypotheses about man and culture and, ultimately, one particular science of man.[4]

The problem of human nature as it relates to both the physiological and moral attributes of man has long been the subject of philosophical and scientific controversy. Thus, the nature versus nurture debate has been a subject of interest for scholars of many disciplinary persuasions.

**This a shortened version of the author's paper given at the Third National Caring Conference.*
†No distinction is made with respect to gender in this paper.

The view that man is a product of his environment, as stated by Hippocrates in *Air, Waters, and Places,* has long been influential. Locke, Rousseau, and other exponents of the nurture theory of human development asserted that the newborn child is but a *tabla rasa,* a blank slate on which everything is written up through experience and learning. In a similar spirit Rousseau's contemporary, Helvetius, insisted that intellectually, man is but a product of his education. The utopian visionary Charles Fourier extended this view to state that universities could, with little effort, produce nations of Shakespeares and Newtons. And more than 100 years ago Thomas Huxley asserted, with characteristic vigor, that the newborn baby arrives, not as shopkeeper, duke, or bishop, but as a "mass of undifferentiated pulp", and it is only through the process of education that we can develop its human potential.

In sharp contrast to the proponents of the nurture thesis, Hobbes, Spencer, and assorted social Darwinists subscribed to the notion that nature *qua* heredity determines to a considerable degree the characteristics of the individual. Also, on the basis of very inadequate statistical evidence, Galton concluded that such a genetically based theory accounted for the stratification of British society. In his view judges begot judges, and the working class spawned generations of people who lacked the intellectual equipment necessary for any form of upward social mobility.

The nature-nurture controversy has extended into the twentieth century and has assumed many dimensions. For example Freud believed that the human mind was shaped from birth by enviromental influences which directed development. Of particular importance were those events which took place around the time of birth. Jung looked even further back to the genesis of the collective mind and related the complexities of the human brain to archetypes as old as the human race itself. Perhaps modern "past lives" therapists also look to such archetypes (at a more personal level) in their attempts to come to terms with the problems of the human mind.[5,6]

Most recently, criminology and psychology have entered the nature-nurture debate with probably the most elaborate empirical theories of the deterministic variety. Doubtless we are all familiar with both the XYY chromosome controversy and the Jensenist hersey. In both cases weak evidence and faulty logic of the cause and effect type combine with ideological *Weltanschauungen* to extend science into the social and the moral spheres.[7] Opposing warcries of entrenched "experts" are forever declaring in favor of what seem to be entirely different conclusions. The work of criminologists, perhaps, stands out best as an example of professional (ideologized) reflections on the nature of man. Depending on the fashion of the day, or the fad the researcher succumbed to, criminals had their heads measured, their bodies somatotyped, their personalities and intelligence tested and rated, and in more recent years their genetic composition investigated to discover if there existed a Y-chromosome excess.[8] While there is no time here to engage in a lengthy discussion of the substantive issues in any of these areas, suffice it to say for the present that the biological evidence for criminal and other "deviant" behavior is far from complete. Moreover, what evidence there is, is usually presented in anything but an ethically neutral, *Wertfrei,* culturally detached arena.

Attempts to define the biological basis of human behavior have been numerous. Ethologists have certainly played an important part in sketching out of the "parable of the beast".[9] Ethology may be defined as the scientific study of the species—specific and genetically mediated behavioral patterns of animals and man.

A major figure in European ethology is Tinbergen, a man convinced that human behavior "is *not* qualitatively different from animals."[10] For Tinbergen, all human behavior has underlying, fundamental, innate drives such as sex, aggression, food seeking, and parental instincts. In reference to the intricate relationship between nature and culture, Tinbergen has observed that there are good grounds "for the conclusion that man's limited behavioral adjustability has been outpaced by the culturally determined changes in his social environment, and that this is why man is now a misfit in his own society."[11]

A popularizer of ethology, Lorenz shares Tinbergen's views. However, Lorenz goes further and asserts that over time, domestication combined with culturally determined changes in human ecology, have resulted in what he terms dysfunctions of numerous species, ie, specific preserving action patterns and culturally adaptive normative responses. The full extent of Lorenz's thesis is realized in his major work, *On Aggression.*[12] He notes that there is a significant lag between man's social instincts and his social inhibitions in which man is unable to "keep pace with the rapid developments of traditional culture, particularly material culture." Aggression, he argues, cannot be controlled through phylogenetically-adapted behavioral mechanisms. Man's inventiveness (eg, weapons of war) has extended instinctive aggression into the realm of the cultural, hence rendering innate controlling mechanisms impotent. Moreover, he declares that the influence of *moral strength,* a cultural product, as a controlling factor over instinctive inclinations, may produce conflicts within the individual, thereby producing dysfunctional nervous disorders, disorders characterized by man's seeming inability to integrate human nature and culture.

The biological basis of behavior, and its relationship to culture, has also been explored in rigorous detail by Eibl-Eibesfeldt in his work *Ethology.*[14] In this work, he emphasizes the importance of the conditioning of inherited behavioral patterns. Aggression is seen as dysfunctional, therefore requiring some form of cultural control. Cooperation within the group is seen as an innate human characteristic.

Contemporary ethologists have developed theories which assert the primacy of innate learning dispositions, drives, instincts, and innate releasing mechanisms. These innate factors are seen to influence behavior in quite decisive ways. Culture is seen as *the* critical controlling factor, the superorganic inhibitor of man's animal instincts.

While the above overview is by no means an exhaustive account of ethological work, it may serve to sketch out some of its central themes. Instead of metaphysics we find the tools of biology turned toward the nature of man. The ethological model of man seeks to replace teleological explanations of human nature with an "empirical statement" which points to our innate propensity for love, aggression, caring, and indifference. It seeks scientific explanation for humanism, or its absence.

Enter Sociobiology

What then of sociobiology? Does the growing body of sociobiological theory shed any light on the problem of human nature? Are we by nature altruistic to others only to the extent that they carry the same genes we carry or to the extent that our *niceness,* or *caring* will be reciprocated? Or is altruism a product of cultural development? These are some of the central questions in the sociobiological debate.

First, let us turn our attention to the basic tenets of sociobiology as expounded by such noted figures as Wilson,[1,3] Alexander,[15] Hamilton,[16] Maynard Smith,[17] Trivers,[18] Dawkins,[2] and West-Eberhard.[19] Briefly, these may be summarized thus:

1) Behavior patterns exhibited by all living systems are adaptive within the stream of evolutionary change.
2) Individual fitness, the share of genes that each individual contributes to the next generation, is to be seen as the essential criterion by which to explain the social behavior of man and beast.
3) Through the mechanism of *kin selection,* altruism (which tends to reduce personal fitness) evolves through natural selection.

Of major importance for the present discussion is the third tenet. This is clarified by Wilson, who stated, "If the genes causing the altruism are shared by two organisms because of common descent, and if the altruistic act by one organism increases the joint contribution to the next generation, the propensity to altruism will spread through the gene pool."[1] Evolutionary process demands that all biological organisms maximize their "inclusive fitness". Through the "calculus of blood ties" the human mind is capable of developing "proportionate altruism". This means that knowledge of biological kinship is a *conditio sine qua non* of kinship selection at the cultural level.

Sociobiologists tend to see man's organic nature and culture as separate dichotomous phenomena. Wilson in particular has been emphatic on this point, and has asserted that "the specific details of culture are nongenetic" and "can be decoupled from the biological system and arranged beside it."[1] It is equally important to note that cultural evolution is seen as quite different from biological evolution. The relationship between man's innate nature and culture is posited to be an antagonistic one.

Enter Altruism

We now turn our attention specifically to altrusim and attempt to explicate what the sociobiologists have to say about our genetic predisposition for altruistic behavior. First, a sociobiological definition of altruism:[18]

> Altruistic behavior can be defined as a behavior that benefits another organism, not closely related, while being apparently detrimental to the organism performing the behavior, benefit and detriment being defined in terms of contribution to inclusive fitness.
>
> Moveover:
>
> One human being leaping into water, at some danger to himself, may be said to display altrusitic behavior. If he were to leap in to save his own child, the behavior would not necessarily be an instance of "altruism;" he may merely be contributing to the survival of his own genes in the child. [Note the highly speculative "may merely" of the author.]

The argument was also made by Trivers that models "that attempt to explain altruistic behavior in terms of natural selection are models designed to take the altruism out of altruism."[18] Hamilton, as early as 1964, claimed to have demonstrated that:[16]

> [the] degree of relationship is an important parameter in predicting how selection will operate, and behavior which appears altruistic may, on knowledge of the genetic relationship of the organisms involved, be explicable in terms of natural selection: those genes being selected for that contribute to their own perpetuation, regardless of which individual the genes appear in.[16]

Human Reciprocal Altruism

Reciprocal altruism is a universal phenomenon finding expression in all known cultures. The following types of altruism are widespread:[16]

1) Helping in times of danger (eg, accidents, predation, intra-specific aggression);
2) Sharing food;
3) Helping the sick;
4) Sharing implements; and
5) Sharing knowledge.

Trivers notes that all these types of altruistic behavior "often meet the criterion of small cost to the giver and great benefit to the taker."[18]

There are two things that stand out here. We may raise these by way of questions. Do we daily calculate "coefficients of relatedness" to "significant" others and then determine the extent to which our altruism will maximize their "success," which will in turn "cause our genes to multiply?"[20] Thus:

> A brother or sister has half of our genes and therefore would be more "worthy" of our investment than a cousin (⅛), who is nevertheless more worthy than a stranger."

The second point of importance which elucidates the sociobiologist's position is related to what philosophers of science refer to as *reductionism.* When we reflect on early evolutionists' accounts of altruistic behavior, we find that they largely explained this phenomenon in terms of group benefit. Thus, a functionalist explanation was offered that addressed altruism and ethics at the level of the group rather than at the level of the individual.[21] Sociobiologists,on the other hand, conceive of evolution as competition among genes rather than among groups or individuals.[20] At least one sociobiologist, Dawkins, argued that the problem of evolution is the problem of competiton among genes (the selfish gene) *tout court.* Evolution "is not about my personal survival but about the maximization of my genetic representation in the next generation: my inclusive fitness." Furthermore:[20]

> If I have three offspring and each of them has half of my genes, and if my self-sacrifice can save them, then the genetic basis of self-sacrifice will be selected for them. Since the offspring represent 150% of my genes, those genes which lead to this kind of "altruism" will increase in the population even if I happen to die in the process....This "gene first" perspective can and does, in the hands of the sociobiologists, give rise to a theory of human nature, a theory which deals with topics ranging from nepotism to sex-role differences, and all in terms of evolutionary biology.

The key to all this is *kin selection.* Sociobiologists are quick to point out that early hominid hunter gatherers (as with contemporary Bushman, !Kung San) consisted of banks of close kin. Trivers asserted that it logically follows that kin selection "must often have operated to favor the evolution of some types of altruistic behavior."[22] He never demonstrated this logical cause and effect connection. Indeed, it is on the subject of kinship and kin selection where the sociobiologists clutch at straws. Wilson is particularly weak on this subject. In the writings of the sociobiologists there is a failure to recognize that kinship selection is culturally defined. Culture is the superorganic context wherein kin selection assumes rule-governed dimensions. Sahlins, in a thought provoking attack on sociobiology, reviewed the ethnographic evidence for the presence of "selective pressures" mediated through kinship selection and declared the sociobiologists wanting.[22] He argued that human kinship systems simply do not conform to the predictions of the sociobiologists:

> Each kinship order has its own theory of heredity of shared substance, which is never the gentic theory of modern biology.

Additionally:

> Such human conceptions of kinship may be so far from biology as to exclude all but a small fraction of a person's genealogical connections from the category of close kin...The human systems ordering reproductive success have an entirely different calculus than that predicted by kin selection and *sequitur est,* by an egoistically conceived natural selection.[22]

In 1906 Van Gennep established his distinction between *parente sociale* and *parente physique*. Malinowski applied this distinction to the Australian aborigines and extended it through a redefinition of the whole notion of consanguinity derived from Morgan (1870), who had postulated that kinship was based on "folk knowledge of biological consanguinity."[23] Influenced by Durkheim, Malinowski observed that "consanguinity was a cultural conceptualization, part of a set of collective representations of any society."[24] He said:

> ...consanguinity...is the set of relations involved by the collective ideas under which facts of procreation are viewed in a given society.

This point was reiterated with greater clarity:

> Consanguinity (as a sociological concept) is therefore not the physiological bond of common blood, it is the social acknowledgment and interpretation of it.[24]

Anthropologists generally, and Sahlins in particular, do place sociobiological theories in a questionable light. Clearly ethologists and sociobiologists have failed to identify the dynamic processes of interaction between the genetic substrates and culture. The mechanisms, the biogrammer, remain shrouded in mystery by what the sociobiologists refer to as simply, a lack of data. It is not so much that their deterministic theories are lacking, but rather their claim of the data being more widely gathered and brought to bear on the problem of biological consanguininty. Perhaps, at best, we are looking at a good example of a necessary but not sufficient explanation.

Barkow correctly noted that the findings of the sociobiologists "will *not* involve rigid behaviors tightly linked to genetics."[20] Nor will behaviors be found to be tied to specific substrates. In short, he stated,

> Modern ethological conceptions of human behavior recognize that it varies on a stability/ability dimension rather than being either "innate" ("genetic") or "acquired". All behavior requires interaction with the environment, if for no other reason than that each and every gene requires complex interactions and feedbacks with the environment for its expression. *The link between genetic substrate and most human behavior is probabilistic rather than deterministic.* [Italics by the author.]

Ethologists and sociobiologists present a view of human nature and human behavior that differs little from their views on animal behavior. As do many behavioristic psychologists (eg, Skinner and Watson), they routinely extrapolate from animal to human behavior. It is here that the problem of generalizing from conditioned animal behavior to human symbolic behavior becomes an exercise in "ratomorphy" and, to put it mildly, understates the full range of human potential.

If man has genetic substrates for particular forms of behavior, he also embraces a symbolic universe, a cultural system that has transcended the animal and defined ubiquitous ontology, thereby explaining metaphysical uncertainty. The "parable of the beast" leads to the "divine", and the "great chain of being" must be examined as cultural evolution that has outpaced biological evolution and sets man apart from other animals.

The Idolatry of Evolution

What I have attempted to do thus far is present an overview of sociobiology, and not an exhaustive account of a highly complex and controversial corpus of knowledge and belief. I do not wish to denigrate the biosocial relations established between man and his environment; rather, I hope to elucidate the sociobiological view of human nature, particularly as it relates to altruistic behavior. However, this brief excursion raises a number of important issues, not the least of which is the problem of the philosophy of natural law. Is sociobiology merely new evolutionary theory, or is it a new kind of biometaphysics where something akin to Adam Smith's invisible hand portions out good and evil to selected carriers? Can we reduce human nature to a mathematical probability cloaked in the guise of genetic substrates? Or is there more to *homo sapiens* than this deterministic elaboration of ratomorphic man?

The answers to these questions may best be sought within the cultural context of normal science (in Kuhn's sense). The philosophical status of certain key concepts in biology brings them as close to the soft human sciences as it does to the physico-chemical ones.[26] The fundamental premises of both ethology and sociobiology are not exempt from this complex interrelationship. This statement clearly introduces the concept of ideology.

Historically, we find that in the 17th century significant changes occurred in the realm of scientific explanation. Young has advanced the following observation:[26]

> ...the quantitative handling of data was related to a fundamental shift in the definition of a scientific explanation. The concept of purpose and value—the final "causes" and teleological explanations—which had been central to the Aristotelian view of nature, were banished from the explanations of science (though not from the philosophy of nature).

Qualitative questions directed towards nature sought answers "in terms of matter, motion, and number." The quantification of the qualities became the *modus operandi* of orthodox science. Young comments further:[26]

> In the physico-chemical sciences this list of so-called "primary qualities" (matter, motion, number) has been modified to include some less precise concepts such as force, energy, and fields, but the fundamental paradigm of explanation—the goal of all science—has been to reduce or explain all phenomena in physico-chemical terms. The history of science is routinely described as a progressive approximation to this goal. This is the metaphysical and methodological explanation for the fact that molecular biology is the queen of the biological sciences and the basis on which other biological (including human) sciences seek, ultimately, to rest their arguments. I need hardly say that this has been a rather forlorn goal for much of biology, and the source of a great deal of sheer bluff.

Biological sciences, for the most part, can be located halfway along a continuum ranging from pure mathematics and the physico-chemical at one end to the softest of human sciences at the other.[26] As a result of this middle position we see that biological sciences involve themselves in the philosophical and methodological problems of the social sciences. Biology, as with other harder sciences, is a cognitive system located within the context of a cultural system. Hence, biological paradigms contain built-in values, values derived from culture. It is important to not let the success of molecular biology obscure the fundamental differences between types of biological knowledge. Biology *qua* biology is in need of a metaphysical critique.

It is my contention that the current debate in and on sociobiology is somewhat similar to that found within the context of the 19th century evolutionary debate. During this period it was clear that social and ideological factors "defined the context of the debate at the same time as they determined key issues about the narrowest scientific problem: the precise mechanism of evolutionary change."[26] Within this context we find such diverse interrelated issues as natural theology, utilitarianism, phrenology, historiography, the idea of progress, and positivism, to name but a few. Young's views are apposite here:[26]

> If we follow the thread of the scientific debate it leads from the economic writings of Adam Smith and T. R. Malthus to the theological and ethical works of Paley, to the theological geology of William Buckland and Alan Sedgwick, to the equally theological—but the anti-literalist and anti-evolutionary writings of Charles Lyell, and on to Darwin, Spencer, and Wallace. This debate was closely intertwined with and fed directly into controversies in psychology, physiology, medicine, sociology, anthropology, and genetics, all of which were invoked in debates on "Social Darwinism" and imperialism. *There is not at any point, any clear line on it, and the related theological, social, political, and ideological issues.* [Italics added by the author.]

The extent to which Darwin's ideas fed into political controversy is well documented.[27] This is particularly true of his conception of the role of struggles between man, and between man and environment. Was this struggle, in both areas, an inevitable evolutionary survival strategy, and was it the *sine qua non* of progress? Darwin somehow managed to avoid this debate. Indeed, he steadfastly refused to engage in discussion that fell into any political arena. His co-discoverer of the theory of evolutioin in natural selection did not fare so well. Wallace, like Darwin, drew upon the work of Malthus and his theory of population, but very soon he became acutely aware that Malthusian theory came into direct conflict with both his philosophy of nature and, more dramatically, with his socialism. As a result of his difficulty with the political implications of Malthusian theory, Wallace abandoned natural selection "as applied to man's physical, mental, and social environment."[27] Moreover, he concluded that the Malthusian population theory was a politically conservative theory drawn upon by liberal and conservative thinkers who attempted to justify their reactionary political philosophies by blaming nature for all the evils of *homo politicus*. Thus, Wallace rightly concluded that conservative thinkers sought explanations for man's inhumanity to man in some inherent property of human nature rather than through analysis of such things as political repression, exploitation, colonial domination, and repressive imperialism. Notions like the survival of the fittest were seen by Wallace as political statements bent on providing *scientific* legitimacy for inequities in and between societies.

Is it possible that we can regard the work of Wilson, Dawkins, Trivers, Lorenz, Jensen, and other proponents of the biodeterministic model of man in the same light? While we must recognize that there are significant differences between these men, they do share an element of biodeterminism in their work, and tend to attribute a biological base to behavior that has a clear sociopolitical (ideological) dimension that cannot be ignored. Should there be some reasonable evidence to support this contention, and I am convinced that there is, then it would not be the first time that science has been selectively drawn upon to support political philosophy or to influence social policy. Spencer, for example, was clear about the place of ideology in his own view of the mechanisms of evolution.[26] He looked to biology to support his extreme version of laissez-faire social theory, and Lamarkianism seemed to hold the answer.[26,28] In a debate with Weismann, where he was defending the inheritance of acquired characteristics, he concluded that "a right answer to the question whether acquired characters are or are not inherited, underlies right beliefs, not only in biology and psychology, but also in education, ethics, and politics."[26]

Huxley, a major supporter of Darwin, in a lecture entitled "Evolution and Ethics" (delivered at Oxford in 1893), put forward a defense of biology which moved away from simply rejecting a fundamental theological view of life "to earnestly advocating that men realize that science and evolutionary theory could not provide a guarantee of progress or a substitute for moral and political discourse." As Young said:[26]

> In the meantime evolution had been invoked to support all sorts of political and ideological positions from the most reactionary to the most progressive, from total *laissez-faire* to revolutionary Marxism. The fallacy which Huxley was combating was the naturalistic one. While agreeing that we cannot infer human morals, much less inevitable social progress, from science, we should not fail to see the complementary point that moral and political views were already deeply embedded *in* the science of the day.

This leads me to the current debate—the question of our genetic predisposition to care—our altruistic substrates. Sociobiologists and ethologists cannot be fully understood unless one is aware of their idolatrous commitment to evolution as both the ultimate context and moving force of human nature: Theirs is a quasi-religious attitude towards Darwinism. Fromm's comments are apposite here:[13]

> The deep need of man not to feel lost and lonely in the world had, of course, been

previously satisfied by the concept of a God who had creted this world and was concerned with each and every creature. When the theory of evolution destroyed the picture of God, as the supreme Creator, confidence in God as the all powerful Father of man fell with it, although many were able to combine a belief in God with the acceptance of the Darwinian theory. But for many of those for whom God was dethroned, the need for a godlike figure did not disappear. Some proclaimed a new god, Evolution, and Darwin as a prophet.

Among the ethologists, Lorenz serves to illustrate this quasi-religious attitude towards Darwinism, although he certainly is not alone in this regard. His use of the term the "great constructors", referring to selection and mutation, resembles the Christian focus on God's acts as moving forces. This is particularly apparent when he uses the singular and refers to the great constructor.[12] This idolatrous quality in Lorenz's work is exemplified in the concluding paragraph of *On Aggression:*[12]

> We know that in the evolution of vertebrates, the bond of personal love and friendship was the epoch-making invention created by the great constructors when it became necessary for two or more individuals of an aggressive species to live peacefully together and to work for a common end. We know that human society is built on the foundation of this bond, but we have to recognize the fact that the bond has become too limited to encompass all that it should: it prevents aggression only between those who know each other and are friends, while obviously it is all active hostility between all men of all nations or ideologies that must be stopped. The obvious conclusion is that love and friendship should embrace all humanity, that we should love all our human brothers indiscriminately. This commandment is not new. Our reason is quite able to understand its necessity as our feeling is able to appreciate its beauty, but nevertheless, *made as we are, we are unable to obey it.* We can feel the full, warm emotion of friendship and love only for individuals, and the utmost exertion of willpower cannot alter this fact. But the great constructors can, and *I believe* they will. *I believe* in the power of human reason, as *I believe* in the power of natural selection. *I believe* that reason can and will exert a selection pressure in the right direction. *I believe* that this, in the not too distant future, will endow our descendants with the faculty of fulfilling the greatest and most beautiful of all commandments.

For Lorenz, the great constructors are to do what God has failed to do. The great constructor is presumably the ultimate *deus ex machina* in this scenario. Wilson, and other sociobiologists, share this view but place their faith in scientific materialism—what they consider to be the true Promethean spirit of science and man. The evolutionary epic has become a secular theology; faith is shown in the following paragraph:[3]

> Human genetics is now growing quickly along with all other branches of Science. In time much knowledge concerning the genetic foundations of social behavior will accumulate, and techniques may become available for altering gene complexes by molecular engineering and rapid selection through cloning. At the very least slow evolutionary change will be feasible through conventional engenics. The human species can change its own nature. What will it choose? Will it remain the same, teetering on a jerrybuilt foundation of partly obsolete Ice-Age

> adaptations? Or will it press on toward still higher intelligence and creativity, accompanied by a greater-or-lesser-capacity for emotional resposne? New patterns of sociality could be installed in bits and pieces. It might be possible to imitate genetically the more nearly perfect nuclear family of the white-handed gibbon or the harmonious sisterhood of the honeybees.

Wilson stated the above in a chapter entitled "Hope". His hope had been expressed much earlier and may be seen as the latest development in a line of thought that gained momentum in the work of the early social Darwinists, who firmly believed in the Idea of Progress.* Condorcet, Comte, Spencer, and others shared Wilson's hope for the future of man. Only the mechanism of progress has changed from the macro-evolution of the earlier social Darwinism to the micro, molecular dimensions of contemporary genetic social evolution of Wilson and his ilk. Bury's remarks seem to hold today:[29]

> Enough has been said to show that the Progress of humanity belongs to the same order of ideas as Providence or personal immortality. It is true or it is false, and like them it cannot be proved either true or false. Belief in it is an act of faith.

I stated at the outset that our philosophy of human nature, the "image of man at the center" shapes our science of man. The parable of the beast as it unfolds in the hands of the new biologists forces us to take issue with their conception of human nature.

Conclusion

Our concern with human caring, our desire to operationalize human altruism, and to understand it, and thereby engage in our essential humanity, is to share a vision of man's ultimate nature. At present we can opt for a number of perspectives drawn from theology, economics, philosophy, politics, biology, anthropology, sociology, psychology, and the harder sciences. The fact that we can choose is to be taken seriously.

As an anthropologist I am interested in cultural diversity. And, as I look around me I see a wide variety of beliefs concerning the nature of man. Such beliefs are the stuff of anthropology. My concern is not so much with the Apollonian promises of genetically encoded behavior, real or imagined, but rather with the choices that make us human. It is these choices, made within a multiplicity of cosmological systems, which serve to elucidate the nature of man generally and human caring specifically. Man's morality was created by reason. Human genes have surrendered their primacy in human evolution to culture, and, to paraphrase Dobzhansky, while our genes may predispose us to speak, they do not tell us what to say.

---

*Apologies to Darwin. This is actually is misnomer. See Hofstader R: *Social Darwinsim in American Thought.* Boston, Beacon Press, 1955. For an earlier statement, see Bury JB: *The Idea of Progress.* London, McMillan, 1920.

References

1. Wilson EO: Sociobiology: The New Synthesis. Harvard University Press, 1975, pp 4, 560.
2. Dawkins R: The Selfish Gene. New York, Oxford University Press, 1976.
3. Wilson EO: On Human Nature. New York, Bantam Books, 1978, p 216.
4. Becker E: Angel in Armor: A Post Freudian Perspective on the Nature of Man. New York, George Braziller, 1969.
5. Dubos, R: So Human an Animal. New York, Charles Scriber's Sons, 1968.
6. Hampson N: The Enlightenment. New York, Pelican Books, 1969.
7. Rex, J: Race, Colonialism and the City. London, Routledge, and Kegan Paul, 1973, pp 230-240.
8. West DJ (ed): Criminological Implications of Chromosome Abnormalities. Cambridge, Institute of Criminology, 1969.
9. Bleibtreu JN: The Parable of the Beast. New York, Bollier Books, 1969.
10. Tinbergen N: The Study of Instinct. New York, Oxford University Press, 1951, p 205.
11. Friedrich (ed): Man and Animal: Studies in Behavior. New York, St. Martin's Press, 1973, p 127.
12. Lorenz K: On Aggression. New York, Harcourt Brace & Jovanovich, 1966.
13. Fromm E: The Anatomy of Human Destructiveness. CT, Fawcett Crest Books, 1973.
14. Eibl-Eibesfeldt I: Ethology: The Biology of Behavior. New York, Holt Reinhart & Winston, 1975.
15. Alexander R: The Search for an evolutionary philosophy of man. In Proceedings of the Royal Society (Victoria), 1971, pp 99-120.
16. Hamilton WD: The genetic evolution of social behavior. Journal of Theoretical Biology, 1964, pp 57-91.
17. Smith JM: On Evolution. Edinburgh, Edinburgh University Press, 1972.
18. Trivers R: The evolution of reciprocal altrusim. Quarterly Review of Biology, 1971, pp 35-37.
19. West-Eberhard MJ: The evolution of social behavior. Quarterly Review of Biology, 1971, pp 35-37.
20. Barkow J: Culture and Sociobiology. American Anthropologist 1:5-6, 14, 1978.
21. cf: Waynne-Edwards VC: Ecology the evolution of social ethics. In Pringle JWS (ed): Biology and the Human Sciences. Oxford, Clarendon Press, 1972, pp 44-69; Flew A: Evolutionary Ethics. London, McMillan, 1967; Pugh GE: The Biological Origin of Human Values New York, Basic Books, 1977; and Stent G: Structural Ethics. The Hasting's Center Report, 1976, pp 32-40.
22. Sahlis M: The Uses and Abuses of Biology: An Anthropological Critique of Sociobiology. Ann Arbor, University of Michigan Press, 1976, p 57.
23. Buchler IR, Selby HA: Kinship and Social Organization: An Introduction to Theory and Method. New York, MacMillian Co, 1968, pp 3-4.
24. Malinowski R: The Family among the Australian Aborigines. New York, Schoekine Books, 1965.
25. Durham W: Towards a coevolutionary theory of Human Biology and Culture. Presented at the 75th Annual Meeting of the AmericanAnthropologicalAssociation, Washington, DC.
26. Young RM: Evolutionary Biology and Ideology: Then and Now. In Fueller, W (ed): The social impact of Modern Biology. London, Routledge & Kegan Paul, 1971, pp 199-214.
27. Eisley L: Darwin's Century: Evolution and The Men Who Discovered It. New York, Anchor Paperbacks, 1959.
28. Rummey J: Herbert Spencer's Sociology. New York, Atherton Press, 1966.
29. Bury JB: The Idea of Progress. London, McMillian, 1920, p 4.

Subject Index

A

B

C

D

E

F

G

H

U

V

W

Author Index